Care of the Patient with Hepatitis C Virus Infection

Editor

BARBARA H. MCGOVERN

INFECTIOUS DISEASE CLINICS OF NORTH AMERICA

www.id.theclinics.com

Consulting Editor
HELEN W. BOUCHER

December 2012 • Volume 26 • Number 4

ELSEVIER

1600 John F. Kennedy Blvd., Suite 1800, Philadelphia, PA 19103-2899.

http://www.theclinics.com

INFECTIOUS DISEASE CLINICS OF NORTH AMERICA Volume 26, Number 4
December 2012 ISSN 0891–5520, ISBN-13: 978-1-4557-4899-0

Editor: Stephanie Donley
Developmental Editor: Teia Stone

Infectious Disease Clinics of North America (ISSN 0891–5520) is published in March, June, September, and December by Elsevier Inc., 360 Park Avenue South, New York, NY 10010-1710. Periodicals postage paid at New York, NY and additional mailing offices. Subscription prices are $271.00 per year for US individuals, $463.00 per year for US institutions, $134.00 per year for US students, $321.00 per year for Canadian individuals, $573.00 per year for Canadian institutions, $383.00 per year for international individuals, $573.00 per year for international institutions, and $185.00 per year for Canadian and international students. To receive student rate, orders must be accompanied by name of affiliated institution, date of term, and the *signature* of program/residency coordinator on institution letterhead. Orders will be billed at individual rate until proof of status is received. Foreign air speed delivery is included in all *Clinics* subscription prices. All prices are subject to change without notice. **POSTMASTER**: Send address changes to *Infectious Disease Clinics of North America*, Elsevier Health Sciences Division, Subcription Customer Service, 3251 Riverport Lane, Maryland Heights, MO 63043. **Customer Service: 1-800-654-2452 (US). From outside of the US and Canada, call 1-314-447-8871. Fax: 1-314-447-8029. E-mail: JournalsCustomerService-usa@elsevier.com (print support) or JournalsOnlineSupport-usa@elsevier.com (online support).**

Infectious Disease Clinics of North America is also published in Spanish by Editorial Inter-MÅdica, Junin 917, 1ᵉʳ A 1113, Buenos Aires, Argentina.

Reprints. For copies of 100 or more, of articles in this publication, please contact the Commercial Reprints Department, Elsevier Inc., 360 Park Avenue South, New York, New York 10010-1710. Tel. (212) 633-3812, Fax: (212) 462-1935, E-mail: reprints@elsevier.com.

Infectious Disease Clinics of North America is covered in *MEDLINE/PubMed (Index Medicus), Current Contents/Clinical Medicine, Science Citation Alert, SCISEARCH,* and *Research Alert.*

Printed and bound by CPI Group (UK) Ltd, Croydon, CR0 4YY

Transferred to digital print 2012

Contributors

CONSULTING EDITOR

HELEN W. BOUCHER, MD, FIDSA, FACP
Director, Infectious Diseases Fellowship Program; Associate Professor of Medicine, Division of Geographic Medicine and Infectious Diseases, Tufts Medical Center, Boston, Massachusetts

GUEST EDITOR

BARBARA H. MCGOVERN, MD
Associate Professor, Tufts University School of Medicine, Director, Viral Hepatitis Clinic, Lemuel Shattuck Hospital, Boston, Massachusetts

AUTHORS

MUHAMMAD SHOAIB AFRIDI, MD
Saint Michael's Medical Center, Newark, New Jersey

PABLO BARREIRO, MD, PhD
Department of Infectious Diseases, Hospital Carlos III, Madrid, Spain

CHRISTOPH T. BERGER, MD
Ragon Institute of Massachusetts General Hospital, Massachusetts Institute of Technology and Harvard Medical School, Boston, Massachusetts; Departments of Internal Medicine and Biomedicine, University Hospital Basel, Basel, Switzerland

HARJIT BHOGAL, MD
Division of Gastroenterology, Hepatology and Nutrition, Virginia Commonwealth University, Richmond, Vermont

CHRISTOPH BOESECKE, MD
Department of Internal Medicine I, Bonn University Hospital, Bonn, Germany

JENNIFER Y. CHEN, MD
Department of Medicine, Brigham and Women's Hospital, Boston, Massachusetts

RAYMOND T. CHUNG, MD
GI Unit, Massachusetts General Hospital, Boston, Massachusetts

JOSÉ VICENTE FERNÁNDEZ-MONTERO, MD, PhD
Department of Infectious Diseases, Hospital Carlos III, Madrid, Spain

JENNIFER A. FLEMMING, MD
Department of Medicine, Viral Hepatitis Center, University of California, San Francisco, California

ELIOT GODOFSKY, MD
Director, University Hepatitis Center, Bradenton, Florida

STUART C. GORDON, MD
Professor of Medicine, Wayne State University School of Medicine; Director of Gastroenterology-Hepatology, Henry Ford Health System, Detroit, Michigan

SYED-MOHAMMED JAFRI, MD
Medical Director Multivisceral Transplantation, Division of Gastroenterology-Hepatology, Henry Ford Health System, Detroit, Michigan

ERIN T. JENKINS, MD
Section of Gastroenterology, Hepatology, and Nutrition, Fellow, University of Chicago Medical Center, Chicago, Illinois

DONALD M. JENSEN, MD
Professor of Medicine, Center for Liver Diseases, Director, University of Chicago Medical Center, Chicago, Illinois

ARTHUR Y. KIM, MD
Assistant Professor of Medicine, Division of Infectious Diseases, Massachusetts General Hospital, Harvard Medical School, Boston, Massachusetts

PABLO LABARGA, MD, PhD
Department of Infectious Diseases, Hospital Carlos III, Madrid, Spain

ANDREW J. MUIR, MD, MHS
Associate Professor of Medicine, Division of Gastroenterology, Duke Clinical Research Institute, Duke University School of Medicine, Durham, North Carolina

JÜRGEN KURT ROCKSTROH, MD
Department of Internal Medicine I, Bonn University Hospital, Bonn, Germany

JIHAD SLIM, MD
Chief of Infectious Disease, Saint Michael's Medical Center, Newark; Program Director Infectious Disease Fellowship, Seton Hall University, West Orange, New Jersey

VINCENT SORIANO, MD, PhD
Department of Infectious Diseases, Hospital Carlos III, Madrid, Spain

RICHARD K. STERLING, MD, MSc
Professor of Medicine, Chief of Hepatology, Division of Gastroenterology, Hepatology and Nutrition, Virginia Commonwealth University, Richmond, Vermont

NORAH A. TERRAULT, MD, MPH
University of California, San Francisco, California

EUGENIA VISPO, MD
Department of Infectious Diseases, Hospital Carlos III, Madrid, Spain

HEINER WEDEMEYER, MD
Department of Gastroenterology, Hepatology and Endocrinology, Hannover Medical School, Hannover, Germany

DAVID L. WYLES, MD
Associate Professor of Medicine, Division of Infectious Diseases, University of California, San Diego, La Jolla, California

Contents

Hepatitis C virus (HCV) has evolved into a true infectious disease that needs the increased involvement of infectious disease (ID) physicians. HCV is a serious public health concern requiring screening, education, reduction of disease transmission, and access to care. Patients coinfected with HCV/human immunodeficiency virus need their ID physicians to be more involved in HCV care and the unique challenges that exist in this patient population. HCV patients overall need more provider resources with expertise. The era of direct-acting antivirals for HCV is creating the need and opportunity for ID physicians to assume an active role in this disease.

It is important to assess the stage of liver fibrosis in chronic hepatitis C to guide treatment decisions. Liver biopsy has limitations in staging fibrosis. Several blood tests, algorithms, and imaging tests have been studied as noninvasive markers to stage fibrosis in hepatitis C. In patients without suspicion for cirrhosis, 2 noninvasive methods can be used to predict presence of absence of significant liver fibrosis; however, liver biopsy remains the gold standard. It is imperative not to miss the diagnosis of cirrhosis, because this has further implications for screening of hepatocellular carcinoma and varices.

Genome-wide association studies have identified polymorphisms located near the gene encoding IL28B, which turned out to be the best predictor of response to pegylated interferon plus ribavirin for chronic hepatitis C virus (HCV) genotype 1 infection. This association was extended to spontaneous clearance of HCV, suggesting shared mechanisms of treatment and natural control of this virus. In addition to the biologic implications for innate immunity and HCV, a variety of clinical studies have suggested possible translation to a useful genetic test for practitioners. This article reviews the discovery, biology, and potential clinical applications that have stemmed from the seminal observation that IL28B polymorphisms are a main predictor of HCV clearance.

> Chronic hepatitis C is a leading cause of clinical complications and mortality in individuals infected with human immunodeficiency virus (HIV). Approval for the first direct-acting antiviral (DAA) against the hepatitis C virus (HCV) has been eagerly awaited for treating patients coinfected with HIV/HCV. The use of first-generation HCV protease inhibitors is challenged by complicated dosing schedules, frequent serious toxicities, unwanted drug interactions, drug resistance, and high cost. First-generation DAAs will eventually be replaced by more potent, well-tolerated, and convenient agents. HIV/HCV co-infection will become restricted to individuals without proper access to health care.

> Recent advances in understanding of the molecular characteristics of the hepatitis C virus have led to the development of novel antiviral therapeutics. Direct-acting antivirals are designed to inhibit viral targets, whereas host-targeted antivirals block host factors that are used by the virus for its own life cycle. The rapid development of agents in multiple classes has led to the promise of shorter therapy duration, an improved side effect profile, and eventually interferon-sparing regimens. This article reviews novel hepatitis C virus therapeutics in development, including mechanism of action, efficacy, and adverse effects.

> The addition of hepatitis C virus NS3 protease inhibitors to interferon-based regimens has dramatically improved response rates. Despite these improvements treatment is now more complex, associated with increased side effects, and has the potential to select resistant variants in those who are not cured. This article discusses the virologic underpinnings for the development of hepatitis C virus–resistant variants (with a focus on telaprevir and boceprevir) and their impact on therapeutic success. Interim guidance on the use of resistance testing and management is provided based on the limited data. Finally, resistance considerations for other classes of inhibitors and the rapidly approaching interferon-free therapeutics regimens are offered.

> The clinical manifestations of cirrhotic liver disease encompass a broad spectrum of conditions that reflect the consequence of high portal pressures that result from fibrosis and diminished hepatic synthetic reserve. Patients with cirrhosis are at heightened risk for the development of

infection, and although the use of prophylactic antimicrobial therapy may be considered lifesaving in the setting of gastrointestinal hemorrhage, there remains controversy regarding such therapy in the management of cirrhotic ascites. The infectious disease specialist is now becoming familiarized with the management of viral hepatitis, which includes screening for hepatocellular carcinoma and vigilance for infectious complications of antiviral therapy.

Christoph Boesecke, Heiner Wedemeyer, and Jürgen Kurt Rockstroh

The first 6 months after exposure to hepatitis C virus (HCV) are regarded as acute hepatitis C (AHC). Two patient populations worldwide share the highest prevalence of AHC virus infection: injection drug users and HIV-positive men who have sex with men. Diagnosis of AHC is often difficult in both patient populations as the acute inflammatory phase can be clinically asymptomatic and patients at highest risk for acquiring AHC (injection drug users) tend to evade regular medical care. This article addresses similarities and differences in the epidemiology, diagnosis, and management of AHC monoinfection and coinfection.

INFECTIOUS DISEASE CLINICS
OF NORTH AMERICA

Preface

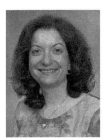

Barbara H. McGovern, MD
Guest Editor

Although the development of effective HIV therapeutics has spanned about 25 years to date, the hepatitis C virus (HCV) therapeutic armamentarium is galloping at lightning speed. About 15 years ago, ribavirin was added to interferon and increased overall viral eradication rates from about 5% to 28% for HCV genotype 1 infection. That was considered a landmark development at the time. The subsequent introduction of the long-acting pegylated interferons increased the overall response rate for difficult to treat genotype 1 infections to just over 50%—again another stellar development. However, with the emergence of the new specifically targeted antiviral medications for HCV, cure rates with triple and quadruple therapies are now surpassing 80% to 90%. Furthermore, interferon-free regimens are now tangible with promising data emerging with multiple classes of drugs, such as the protease inhibitors, NS5A inhibitors, polymerase inhibitors, and other agents.

So, the armamentarium is near at hand, but the number of HCV-knowledgeable clinicians is limited. Furthermore, the number of patients who are diagnosed with HCV is going to increase greatly over the next few years due to expanded HCV screening among persons born from 1945 to 1965, as recommended by the Centers for Disease Control in August 2012. It is estimated that approximately 800,000 persons in the United States do not know they are infected. This low rate of awareness is partly due to failures of screening policies based on risk. Patients often do not want to discuss potential past risks with their medical provider due to concerns regarding stigma. With a universal screening approach of this birth cohort, stigma will be averted and hopefully case findings will be augmented since this older segment of the US population is at risk for liver-related morbidity and mortality.

But screening and diagnosis are not enough. Clinicians who are well-versed in the art of combination antiviral therapy are needed to take on the many patients with advanced fibrosis before the complications of cirrhosis and end-stage liver disease ensue. Infectious disease clinicians are well-poised for this task but need to fully understand the implications of advanced liver disease and the significant adverse events associated with the approved triple therapies in the clinic today, including pegylated interferon, ribavirin, plus approved HCV protease inhibitors, boceprevir or telaprevir. Although current therapies are associated with a myriad of potential adverse events,

Infect Dis Clin N Am 26 (2012) xi–xii
http://dx.doi.org/10.1016/j.idc.2012.08.013
0891-5520/12/$ – see front matter © 2012 Elsevier Inc. All rights reserved.

many patients will not be able to wait for what promises to be simpler and better tolerated regimens.

Within this supplement of the *Infectious Disease Clinics of North America*, we bring a collection of articles by the most outstanding hepatologists and infectious disease experts in the world. You, the reader, will reap the benefit of years of clinical expertise covering the evaluation and staging of liver disease, approach to the treatment naïve and treatment-experienced patient, care of the patient with cirrhosis, the latest antiviral agents, concepts on HCV drug resistance, and finally, the approach to special patient populations, such as the HIV-infected patient with HCV-related liver disease. This outstanding supplement promises to bridge any knowledge gaps that you may have as you take on the challenge of creating a healthier society where HCV will hopefully become an infection of the past.

Barbara H. McGovern, MD
Tufts University School of Medicine
Viral Hepatitis Clinic
Lemuel Shattuck Hospital
Jamaica Plain, MA 02130, USA

E-mail address:
bmcgovern@tuftsmedicalcenter.org

Why Should Infectious Disease Physicians Care for the Hepatitis C–Infected Patient?

Eliot Godofsky, MD

KEYWORDS

- Hepatitis C • HIV/HCV coinfection • Liver biopsy • Access to care • Birth cohort
- Treatment bottleneck

KEY POINTS

- The volume of persons diagnosed with hepatitis C virus (HCV) will be increasing.
- HCV therapy is improving rapidly, but with additional complexity.
- Options for patient care have become limited.
- There is an increasing need for more physician involvement in HCV care.
- Infectious disease physicians are ideally suited for HCV care.

HEPATITIS C: A LIVER DISEASE OR INFECTIOUS DISEASE?

The agent known as non-A, non-B hepatitis was formally characterized as hepatitis C virus (HCV) in 1989.[1,2] Effective antibody screening virtually eliminated HCV from the national blood supply in the United States by 1992. Before this time, there was little known about the true scope of the HCV epidemic, the natural history of the disease, long-term consequences of infection, or the types of therapeutic options required. Patient care was largely observational, supportive, and primarily in the hands of hepatologists. However, these discoveries firmly established that a historical liver disease was also a traditional infectious disease with all the trimmings.

Treatment emerged in 1991 with Food and Drug Administration approval of the first α-interferon for chronic HCV. Sustained virologic response (SVR) rates were low, at 7% to 11% in patients with genotype 1, and 29% to 33% in patients with genotypes 2 and 3.[3,4] Response to therapy was initially based on transaminase reduction, and later replaced by qualitative and quantitative viral parameters. Patient tolerance of interferon therapy was challenging from the onset, with high discontinuation rates commonly encountered. Efficacy improved dramatically with the addition of ribavirin to interferon in 1998 and subsequent approvals of pegylated interferons by 2002, boosting response rates to 45% in patients with genotype 1 and 75% in patients with genotypes 2 and 3.[5,6]

University Hepatitis Center, 6010 Pointe West Boulevard, Bradenton, FL 32409, USA
E-mail address: egodofsky@gmail.com

Infect Dis Clin N Am 26 (2012) 839–847
http://dx.doi.org/10.1016/j.idc.2012.08.001
id.theclinics.com

Outcomes with human immunodeficiency virus (HIV)/HCV-coinfected patients were typically poor with initial interferon regimens, improving to 29% with pegylated interferon/ribavirin combination therapy in patients with genotype 1.[7]

During this period of initial drug development and expanding therapeutic options, relatively few infectious disease (ID) specialists were engaged in day-to-day HCV care. Although some ID physicians were involved in research on HCV epidemiology, transmission, and HIV/HCV coinfection, the vast majority of evaluation, treatment, and clinical research was a hepatology effort.

What is so different about HCV? Why such a departure from the "point guard" role the ID physician assumes in HIV care? The unique challenges of coinfected HIV patients cannot be the only reason. On first blush, the answers may appear intuitive when considering the relationship of HIV to the ID physician:

- HIV (a sexually transmitted disease) was an established public health concern
- Monitoring involves assessment of the immune system
- Care is primarily office-based and rarely involves procedures
- Management includes prescribing multiple antiviral agents
- Most complications are infections
- Providers commonly assumed primary care for their patients

By contrast, HCV as a "liver disease," was characterized by:

- An emerging public health concern
- Monitoring based on liver-function tests
- Complications primarily liver-related
- Liver biopsy needed to "stage" and follow disease progression
- Endoscopic procedures and liver imaging
- Few therapeutic options
- Liver transplantation possibility

Initially these 2 viruses seemed to have found different homes for different reasons. My experience has been that "authorship" of the liver biopsy and the potential complications of end-stage liver disease were the primary considerations in directing patients to hepatology. I have never completely understood nor reconciled why this was the standard case. A liver biopsy is a means to an end, not unlike a CD4 count is for staging an HIV patient. Hepatologists, interventional radiologists, and surgeons perform liver biopsies, followed by the histologic assessment of inflammation and fibrosis. It is the interpretation of this information that governs prognosis and justifies treatment recommendations. Familiarity and understanding of the data should be the key requisites, not the mechanism of acquisition. In addition, the advent of noninvasive markers of fibrosis, elastography, and therapies of increased tolerability and efficacy are likely to relegate liver biopsies to the exception rather than the rule. Although management of liver-related morbidity clearly requires expertise in hepatology, significant complications (liver failure, hepatoma, encephalopathy, bleeding, and so forth) are relatively uncommon in patients without cirrhosis, and vigilance for their development is a skill the ID physician can equally employ.

In 1995, I treated a patient with well-controlled HIV, active HCV, and significant fibrosis on liver biopsy with interferon monotherapy. The community where I practice had little experience with HCV, and published treatment of HIV/HCV coinfection was mostly anecdotal. I did some research, followed the therapy algorithm, and treated the patient for 48 weeks. He did surprisingly well, obtained an SVR, and remains HCV-free to this day. We all start with our first patient. Less than a year later, I became an investigator in the interferon/ribavirin registration trials. A letter was sent to all physicians in my community notifying them of a new treatment available for HCV. Within 6 months, I witnessed a deluge of referrals and rapidly became the primary HCV provider in my area. This situation has not changed in over 15 years. At the beginning, I was often the only ID physician at various HCV meetings and conferences I attended, but found colleagues who both educated me and welcomed my perspective. I do not perform liver biopsies myself; I have acquired a reasonable appreciation of the needs of patients with advanced liver disease, know how to screen for hepatoma, ask for assistance from my liver colleagues when appropriate, and refer patients to the transplant center when indicated. For my practice and my patients, this has evolved into a very comfortable dynamic. While I continue to treat my population of coinfected patients and participate in clinical trials, care of monoinfection is the staple of my HCV practice. This manner of work has developed from traditional ID training, some good HIV experience, and an interest in addressing an unmet medical need in my community.

So if we accept that HCV has a dual nature, why have things developed so unilaterally from a provider perspective, and should this continue to be the case? Other specialties certainly treat many common and complex infectious diseases, asking for additional guidance when appropriate. However, I think HCV inherently represents a different scenario related to the high HCV rate in HIV patients, and the unique aspects of supply and demand evolving with HCV care. Because our HIV patients benefit from the skills of their physicians in a multidisciplinary approach to care, why not apply the model to HCV, coinfected and/or monoinfected? By examining a few important factors, we can see why the opportunity now exists for ID physicians to become more involved in a disease that lends itself to our expertise and needs our help.

FEW HCV PATIENTS RECEIVE TREATMENT

Hepatitis C is a curable disease with durable SVR demonstrated in more than 99% of patients.[8] Successful therapy is associated with decreased liver-related morbidity and mortality, decreased all-cause mortality, decreased need for transplantation, cost-effectiveness in terms quality life years preserved, decreased costs to the health care system, and a reduction in the pool of infected persons.[9-13] Patients view cure of HCV like a dream come true, with physician and office staff satisfaction not lagging far behind. However, despite these and other achievements likely to increase with expanded direct antiviral therapy (DAA) therapy, why have so few patients been treated, and can ID physicians help improve this situation moving forward?

A 2009 analysis demonstrated that from 2002 to 2007, new prescriptions for HCV declined by 30%, and by the end of 2007 only 21% of all estimated infected persons had cumulatively received antiviral therapy.[14] Projections indicated that only 14.5% of liver-related deaths due to HCV during 2002 to 2030 would be prevented if this trend continued.[15] This perplexing and discouraging state of affairs can be traced to several factors[15-19]:

- At-risk individuals unaware of infection
- Physician and patient misperceptions concerning the need for referral and treatment efficacy
- Patient factors such as advanced disease, concurrent medical problems, drug contraindications, asymptomatic status, perceived need for liver biopsy, and lifestyle
- High discontinuation rates on therapy
- Low rates of insurance among HCV patients
- Race and HIV coinfection
- The paucity of specialists interested in treating HCV

Some of these barriers to care will be improved with better screening, wider education, and enhanced therapy. It is also unclear as to how much impact more effective protease inhibitor (PI) therapy will have, because of complexity, side effects, cost, and further "warehousing" of patients anticipating even newer therapies. However, expanding the pool of specialists engaged in HCV will be necessary under any circumstance, and represents a critical, rate-determining step in care. Involving more ID physicians will go a long way to achieving this end.

THE VOLUME OF HCV PATIENTS WILL INCREASE OVER THE NEXT DECADE

The current burden of HCV-infected patients will increase over the next decade. The Centers for Disease Control and Prevention estimate that 50% to 75% are unaware of their infection.[20] Recent modeling indicates that more than 800,000 persons with HCV would be diagnosed with one-time "birth cohort" screening of all persons born between 1945 and 1965.[21] These draft recommendations are likely to become formally endorsed later in 2012, and supplement the current risk-based guidelines. Similar modeling indicates that one-time testing of all persons aged 20 to 69 would yield comparable results.[22] Both models demonstrate the cost-effectiveness of expanded screening (in terms of quality life years saved), but would require improved rates of referral, treatment, and cure to be truly impactful.

Although it remains to be seen at what pace new testing recommendations would identify HCV cases, and how quickly these persons would access care, the effects will be significant on an already stressed system.

THE COMPLEXITY AND INTENSITY OF HCV CARE IS STRAINING AVAILABLE PROVIDER RESOURCES

The availability and rapid development of DAA therapy for HCV is changing the entire face of HCV care. From patient and provider perspectives, this situation has engendered both benefits and unexpected challenges:

- More treatment-naïve patients, including those "warehoused" in expectation of new drugs, will want treatment. As DAA therapy moves to all oral-based treatments with higher efficacy, the number of eligible patients will increase even further.
- Previous treatment-failure patients now have options.
- Clinics' resources needed to manage patients on therapy have substantially increased. More staff time is needed for insurance authorizations, patient education, management of side effects and drug interactions, and viral response monitoring. More patients will be on therapy and more total time per patient will be required. Established patients coming back into active care, combined with new patients needing appointments, have fueled the aptly named "HCV referral and treatment bottleneck."[23] Increasing the numbers of diagnosed persons will only intensify this backlog. Hepatologists as the primary HCV providers are the limiting step in the evaluation and treatment part of this process. Long wait times for new and established patients to be seen are increasingly described.[24]
- In a basic business model, increased volume is generally desirable and contributes to financial viability. The economics of HCV care are unfortunately not so typical, with facility overhead relatively high compared with the patient care revenue (a situation common in HIV). Current HCV treatment is substantially more office-resource intensive. My own clinic, used to handling a high volume of active HCV patients, can accommodate about 30% fewer patients on active

PI therapy with the same staff size, and waiting times for new patients are longer. Our hepatology colleagues are finding the highest-volume clinics and offices are the most overwhelmed by a patient load with challenging economics. Shorter treatment courses, and revenue from procedures and clinical trials can partially offset this situation. Smaller-volume and community-based practices are opting out of HCV care with increasing frequency, further transitioning care to the already burdened higher-volume providers. Changes in therapy have created a relatively unique situation whereby the logistics of better therapy actually act as an impediment to the delivery of care.

OPTIONS FOR IMPROVING DELIVERY OF HCV CARE ARE LIMITED

Several strategies have been proposed to optimize resources for HCV care[24–27]:

- Primary care physician (PCP) interventions before referral to specialty care
- PCPs directly providing HCV treatment
- Outreach models
- Triage patients based on disease severity
- Increased use of physician extenders
- Involvement of other specialists

HCV is a chronic disease whereby disease progression typically occurs over years to decades. Despite high levels of patient anxiety after diagnosis, urgent referral to a specialist is rarely indicated. In the meantime, PCPs could initiate education, additional screenings, vaccinations, and lifestyle modifications prior to specialist consultation. Valuable in concept, and high in potential, implementation at this level has been difficult at best, and few patients come referred with such packaging. It is equally difficult to imagine engaging already busy primary doctors and their staff in complex HCV care. An exception has been the success of the ECHO project developed at the University of New Mexico.[24] Using "telehealth" technology, rural PCPs effectively comanaged HCV patients on treatment.

How can established offices handle increasing patient volume? Physician extenders have been an essential and cost-effective element of HCV care for years. Evaluating, educating, and managing patients on therapy, the double-edged sword of new treatments is making their responsibilities greater and their schedules tighter. Could triaging treatment initiation by disease status soften patient volume overload? A system of "distributive justice"[25] would allow the sickest patients to start therapy sooner than patients with mild disease. This solution is a logical one to a medical backlog, and would be unlikely to cause any true harm to patients (other than anxiety). The problem is that many patients, even with proper education, will have a difficult time accepting this concept especially if they have already been waiting for new drugs or new appointments, or fail to understand why having adequate insurance coverage does not guarantee prompt treatment.

The aforementioned options all have varying degrees of merit, and more solutions are likely to be found. Because physicians need to lead these efforts, developing the "perfect match" of HCV and the ID physician, a resource already in place, makes perfect sense, and merits further exploration.[28]

WHY ID PHYSICIANS ARE WELL SUITED TO TREAT HCV

ID physicians possess an excellent skill set that is well suited to many aspects of HCV treatment. A common approach has been to compare HIV care with HCV care, acknowledge the impressive parallels that exist, and apply these concepts and experiences universally.

HCV is a public health concern with an inherent focus on risk-factor identification, diagnosis, preventing transmission, education, and providing access to care; this is familiar ground for ID physicians working closely with public health systems. ID physicians are very experienced at handling sensitive issues with compassion, and we can support health care providers and health care institutions by educating the patients, their significant others, and their families.

Once diagnosed, HCV patients ask familiar questions about sexual transmission, disclosure to friends and family, workplace concerns, and necessary lifestyle changes. Patients often want opinions on herbal therapies, holistic remedies, and alternative health care options, along with or in lieu of medical therapies they may be offered. Patients seek guidance on initiating therapy, waiting for newer drugs, or participating in clinical trials. Most ID physicians have experience and proficiency in this arena. We initiate therapies based on disease status, risk, and natural history projections. We construct complex antiviral regimens, monitoring closely for response and resistance, and change or abandon ineffective therapies. The latter is often the most difficult part of the job. Typical side effects of HCV therapies include such familiar opponents as infection, rashes, depression, anemia, and neutropenia. Substance abuse and psychiatric disease are well-known challenges to patients. ID practices taking on HCV will find the experience of their staff a very valuable asset.

Although many ID physicians are comfortable managing noninfectious medical issues and complications in their patients, it is important to seek expert consultation when the need arises. These critical collaborations will engender the best patient outcomes. I believe that familiarity with conditions specific to the HCV patient as a "liver disease" is essential to providing comprehensive care, but this must be coupled with appropriate hepatology consultation. For example, the ID physician should recognize the necessary surveillance of cirrhotic patients for hepatocellular cancer, and implement scheduled α-fetoprotein levels and imaging studies. If an abnormal result is found, specialist consultation should be sought. The same principles apply to identifying appropriate patients for evaluation in a liver transplant center, before the acute need arises and an important opportunity may be missed. HCV represents a disease eminently amenable to efficient comanagement of patients without engendering unnecessary "turf" battles. Collaboration with our colleagues is a skill at which ID physicians usually excel.

Lastly, it must be borne in mind that some ID physicians have (or will) focus primarily on coinfected patients, others on HCV monoinfected patients, and still others on some mix of the two populations. The particular scenario will be based on patient demographics, practice type, resources, need, and so forth. Developing ID management of coinfection has the obvious advantages of a single provider with expertise related to both viruses. On a per-patient basis alone, this approach would tremendously offload the hepatologists. Physicians developing a comfort level in treating the additional challenges of coinfection often have a smoother transition when taking on care of monoinfected patients. For many of us, this has been the (back) door into broader care of HCV patients.

GETTING PREPARED AND GAINING EXPERIENCE

Continuing medical care and experience will be the key elements in developing expert HCV care. Education should start with ID fellowship programs incorporating HCV in standard curriculums. Options include mentoring within the division, outsourcing rotations to Hepatology, or developing joint rotations for fellows from both divisions. Experiences in caring for coinfected patients in the HIV clinic should also be developed. For physicians already in practice, educational opportunities and peer-reviewed guidance are increasingly available. To this end, the Infectious Disease Society of America (IDSA) has taken a lead role by chartering the Hepatitis Task Force in 2012 with specific goals including guideline development, increasing educational opportunities through the annual meeting and the expanded IDSA Web site, and development of a hepatitis core curriculum for fellowship training. Upcoming annual meetings will feature more hepatitis-related content, interactive sessions, and production of enduring materials. Similar to this issue of *Infectious Disease Clinics*, our society journals have committed to increasing HCV-related content relevant to the practicing clinician. Physicians will also find greater Internet availability of webinars, case studies, slide presentations, and conference reports on Web sites such as Medscape, Clinical Care Options, Practice Point Communications, and those from Johns Hopkins, the International AIDS Society, and the HIV Medical Association. Mentoring at designated HCV centers of excellence is another possibility being explored. There are now many options that can update and prepare ID physicians for HCV care.

INTEGRATING HCV CARE IN INFECTIOUS DISEASE PRACTICES

If you are concerned about having enough patients to build HCV into your practice, expect to experience the "Field of Dreams" effect: "if you build it, they will come." It might also be useful to increase awareness about screening recommendations and new HCV therapies directly to the referring physicians, hospitals, and media outlets in your community. Recently, we distributed a brief memo to all our PCPs reviewing this updated information. The result was a noticeable increase in new HCV diagnoses, and patients (new and previously diagnosed) referred for evaluation. Reaching out to the "silent" numbers of diagnosed patients never properly evaluated, or lost to follow-up, is a challenging but valuable endeavor.

The inclusion of HCV care into a typical office or hospital-based ID practice is unlikely to require much systems modification. Staff may benefit from "in services" related to HCV, and use the tracking tools, patient management assistance, and chart aids available through independent and pharmaceutical company Web sites (ie, www.hep-druginteractions.org). In our center, patients have a specific nursing visit before initiation of therapy covering drug administration, needle disposal, common side effects, standing laboratory orders, and vaccinations. Involvement of family, significant other, or friend is strongly recommended. A well-trained staff and a prepared patient typically produce improved outcomes.

Lastly, mention should be made about the potential value of clinical trials for treatment of HCV. These studies may offer patients variations on standard therapies, newer drugs with more effective or attractive profiles, or salvage options. For financially challenged or uninsured patients needing therapy, clinical trials may offer the only realistic option. For physicians relatively new to HCV, participation in clinical trials gives a structured treatment and management framework to follow. Revenue generated from clinical trials can also help offset the high cost of patient care. Unfortunately, there is currently no federal or universal state funding for HCV treatment (Ryan White Part B covers HCV therapy in HIV patients only).

SUMMARY

HCV may have started life as a liver disease, but it has clearly evolved into a true infectious disease that needs the increased involvement of the ID community. HCV is a serious public health concern that needs our help in screening, education, reduction of disease transmission, and access to care. HCV/HIV-coinfected patients need their ID physicians to be more involved in HCV care and the unique challenges that exist in this patient population. HCV patients as a whole need more provider resources with expertise. The era of direct-acting antivirals for HCV is creating both the need and opportunity for ID physicians to assume an active role in this disease. Time to get started.

REFERENCES

1. Choo QL, Kuo G, Weiner AJ, et al. Isolation of a cDNA clone derived from a blood-borne non-A, non-B viral hepatitis genome. Science 1989;244(4902):359–62.
2. Kuo G, Choo QL, Alter HJ, et al. An assay for circulating antibodies to a major etiologic virus of human non-A, non-B hepatitis. Science 1989;244(4902):362–4.
3. Poynard T, Marcellin P, Lee SS, et al. Randomised trial of interferon alpha2b plus ribavirin for 48 weeks or for 24 weeks versus interferon alpha2b plus placebo for 48 weeks for treatment of chronic infection with hepatitis C virus. International Hepatitis Interventional Therapy Group (IHIT). Lancet 1998;352(9138):1426–32.
4. McHutchison JG, Gordon SC, Schiff ER, et al. Interferon alfa-2b alone or in combination with ribavirin as initial treatment for chronic hepatitis C. Hepatitis Interventional Therapy Group. N Engl J Med 1998;339(21):1485–92.
5. Manns MP, McHutchison JG, Gordon SC, et al. Peginterferon alfa-2b plus ribavirin compared with interferon alfa-2b plus ribavirin for initial treatment of chronic hepatitis C: a randomised trial. Lancet 2001;358(9286):958–65.
6. Fried MW, Shiffman ML, Reddy KR, et al. Peginterferon alfa-2a plus ribavirin for chronic hepatitis C virus infection. N Engl J Med 2002;347(13):975–82.
7. Torriani FJ, Rodriguez-Torres M, Rockstroh JK, et al. Peginterferon alfa-2a plus ribavirin for chronic hepatitis C virus infection in HIV-infected patients. N Engl J Med 2004;351(5):438–50.
8. Swain MG, Lai MY, Shiffman ML, et al. A sustained virologic response is durable in patients with chronic hepatitis C treated with peginterferon alfa-2a and ribavirin. Gastroenterology 2010;139(5):1593–601.
9. Veldt BJ, Heathcote EJ, Wedemeyer H, et al. Sustained virologic response and clinical outcomes in patients with chronic hepatitis C and advanced fibrosis. Ann Intern Med 2007;147(10):677–84.
10. Kasahara A, Tanaka H, Okanoue T, et al. Interferon treatment improves survival in chronic hepatitis C patients showing biochemical as well as virological responses by preventing liver-related death. J Viral Hepat 2004;11(2):148–56.
11. Saab S, Hunt DR, Stone MA, et al. Timing of hepatitis C antiviral therapy in patients with advanced liver disease: a decision analysis model. Liver Transpl 2010;16(6):748–59.
12. Liu S, Cipriano LE, Holodniy M, et al. New protease inhibitors for the treatment of chronic hepatitis C: a cost-effectiveness analysis. Ann Intern Med 2012;156(4):279–90.
13. Backus LI, Boothroyd DB, Phillips BR, et al. A sustained virologic response reduces risk of all-cause mortality in patients with hepatitis C. Clin Gastroenterol Hepatol 2011;9(6):509–516.e1.
14. Volk ML, Tocco R, Saini S, et al. Public health impact of antiviral therapy for hepatitis C in the United States. Hepatology 2009;50(6):1750–5.
15. Volk ML. Antiviral therapy for hepatitis C: why are so few patients being treated? J Antimicrob Chemother 2010;65(7):1327–9.

16. Institute of Medicine. Hepatitis and liver cancer: a national strategy for prevention and control of hepatitis B and C. Washington, DC: The National Academies Press; 2010.

17. Ong JP, Collantes R, Pitts A, et al. High rates of uninsured among HCV-positive individuals. J Clin Gastroenterol 2005;39(9):826–30.

18. Butt AA, Tsevat J, Leonard AC, et al. Effect of race and HIV co-infection upon treatment prescription for hepatitis C virus. Int J Infect Dis 2009;13(4):449–55.

19. Ghany MG, Strader DB, Thomas DL, et al. Diagnosis, management, and treatment of hepatitis C: an update. Hepatology 2009;49(4):1335–74.

20. Mitchell AE, Colvin HM, Palmer Beasley R. Institute of Medicine recommendations for the prevention and control of hepatitis B and C. Hepatology 2010; 51(3):729–33.

21. Rein DB, Smith BD, Wittenborn JS, et al. The cost-effectiveness of birth-cohort screening for hepatitis C antibody in U.S. primary care settings. Ann Intern Med 2012;156(4):263–70.

22. Coffin PO, Scott JD, Golden MR, et al. Cost-effectiveness and population outcomes of general population screening for hepatitis C. Clin Infect Dis 2012; 54(9):1259–71.

23. McGowan CE, Fried MW. Barriers to hepatitis C treatment. Liver Int 2012; 32(Suppl 1):151–6.

24. Arora S, Thornton K, Murata G, et al. Outcomes of treatment for hepatitis C virus infection by primary care providers. N Engl J Med 2011;364(23):2199–207.

25. Aronsohn A, Jensen D. Distributive justice and the arrival of direct-acting antivirals: who should be first in line? Hepatology 2011;53(6):1789–91.

26. Ford N, Singh K, Cooke GS, et al. Expanding access to treatment for hepatitis C in resource-limited settings: lessons from HIV/AIDS. Clin Infect Dis 2012;54(10): 1465–72.

27. Gujral H, Viscomi C, Collantes R. The role of physician extenders in managing patients with chronic hepatitis C. Cleve Clin J Med 2004;71(Suppl 3):S33–7.

28. McGovern BH. HCV and the ID physician: a perfect match. Clin Infect Dis 2012; 55(3):414–7.

Staging of Liver Disease
Which Option is Right for My Patient?

Harjit Bhogal, MD, Richard K. Sterling, MD, MSc*

KEYWORDS

- Hepatitis C • Noninvasive staging • Liver fibrosis

KEY POINTS

- It is important to assess the stage of liver fibrosis in chronic hepatitis C to guide treatment decisions.
- Liver biopsy has limitations in staging fibrosis, including sampling error and intraobserver and interobserver variability.
- Several blood tests, algorithms, and imaging tests have been studied as noninvasive markers to stage fibrosis in hepatitis C.
- In patients without suspicion for cirrhosis, 2 noninvasive methods can be used to predict presence of absence of significant liver fibrosis; however, liver biopsy remains the gold standard.
- It is imperative not to miss the diagnosis of cirrhosis, because this has further implications for screening of hepatocellular carcinoma and varices.

INTRODUCTION

Chronic hepatitis C virus (HCV) affects more than 4 million Americans. HCV can progress to cirrhosis after decades of infection and result in complications related to portal hypertension, including hepatic encephalopathy, development of varices, and ascites. Cirrhosis also increases the risk of hepatocellular carcinoma (HCC). As a result, HCV is the leading indication for liver transplantation. Consequently, the accurate identification of advanced fibrosis in those with HCV is important in the management of infected patients. With recent advances in HCV therapy, identification of those with cirrhosis also affects duration of therapy.

STAGING LIVER DISEASE IN HCV FOR TREATMENT CONSIDERATIONS: CURRENT RECOMMENDATIONS

Until the advent of the direct antiviral agents (DAA), boceprevir and telaprevir, the management of chronic viral hepatitis C included pegylated interferon (PEG-IFN) in

Division of Gastroenterology, Hepatology and Nutrition, Virginia Commonwealth University, Richmond, VA, USA
* Corresponding author. Section of Hepatology, VCU Medical Center, West Hospital, Room 1478, 1200 East Broad Street, Richmond, VA 23298-0341.
E-mail address: rksterli@vcu.edu

Infect Dis Clin N Am 26 (2012) 849–861
http://dx.doi.org/10.1016/j.idc.2012.08.002
0891-5520/12/$ – see front matter © 2012 Elsevier Inc. All rights reserved.

combination with ribavirin. In patients with genotype 2 and 3, a liver biopsy was not often necessary because sustained virologic response (SVR) is 70% to 80% with PEG-IFN and ribavirin compared with 40% to 50% in those with genotype 1. Given the suboptimal response in genotype 1, liver biopsy was often used to identify those with advanced fibrosis who might benefit from therapy and avoid treatment side effects in those with more mild disease.[1] With the advent of triple therapy and higher SVR rates (60%–75%), the recommendations for liver biopsy have now become debatable in those with genotype 1.

THE LIVER BIOPSY IN STAGING HCV: BENEFITS AND RISKS

Histologic assessment of a liver biopsy specimen is the gold standard diagnostic test to assess liver inflammation, fibrosis, and presence of steatosis, which can guide the physician in identifying whether the patient requires treatment more immediately, or whether treatment can be delayed, and perhaps leaving more room for further developments in therapies for HCV. The presence of advanced fibrosis, bridging fibrosis, or cirrhosis indicates that the patient is at an increased risk of hepatic decompensation and HCC, which require periodic surveillance with ultrasound scans and endoscopy for varices.

However, the liver biopsy is an invasive procedure and the risks and benefits should be carefully evaluated. Liver biopsies can be performed either percutaneously via ultrasound guidance at the bedside or through a transjugular approach under fluoroscopy by an interventional radiologist. The transjugular approach also allows measurement of the hepatic vein pressure gradient. Histologic assessment identifies the degree of inflammation, steatosis, and importantly fibrosis.

The risks of undergoing a liver biopsy include pain, bleeding, infection, and perforation.[2–4] Patients with end-stage renal disease and hemophilia may be at higher risk of bleeding, and desmopressin or factors, respectively, are often administered to minimize this risk in these patient populations.[5,6] In addition to the risks of the procedure, there are also limitations of the liver biopsy, including the size of the liver biopsy specimen, interobserver and intraobserver variability in histologic assessment, and sampling error. In a study of liver biopsy samples taken from both the right and left lobes of the liver, there was a difference in inflammation grade in one-quarter of the patients and a difference in fibrosis staging in one-third of patients, showing the significant variability in HCV-related disease, which can be seen within the same individual.[7] Studies of interobserver variability among pathologists have shown good concordance in assessing early or advanced liver disease (ie, portal fibrosis vs cirrhosis). However, when they assessed several other histologic features, there was a wide range of concordance.[8] Intraobserver variability is another limitation of liver biopsy. Various lengths of liver biopsy specimens have been assessed at 5 mm, 10 mm, 15 mm, and greater than 20 mm and as the size of the biopsy specimen is increased there is less intraobserver variability.[9] It has been suggested that liver biopsy specimens for assessment of fibrosis in HCV should be 25 mm long and contain 8 to 10 portal tracts.[10] Therefore, although liver biopsy remains the gold standard, sampling error and interobserver and intraobserver variability in histologic assessment are limitations to accurate grading and staging of liver inflammation and fibrosis.

NONINVASIVE MARKERS OF STAGING LIVER DISEASE

Because of the limitations of liver biopsy and patient acceptance, there has been intense interest in developing accurate noninvasive markers to stage liver disease in

HCV, including blood tests, transient elastography (TE), imaging studies, and breath tests.

Blood Tests

Several routine and nonroutine blood tests have been evaluated in isolation or in combination to identify an optimal biomarker or model to stage liver disease in HCV. Some models use common tests that are readily available, whereas others include more specific tests of collagen production or degradation. The key blood tests and models are discussed in this review. **Table 1** includes a summary of blood tests and models not discussed that have also been studied as biomarkers in staging liver disease in HCV.

Aspartate Aminotransferase/Platelet Ratio Index

The aspartate aminotransferase/platelet ratio index (APRI) was developed and validated as a noninvasive tool to predict fibrosis in HCV.[11] In the retrospective single-center study that developed the APRI, significant fibrosis was defined as an Ishak score of 3 or more, whereas many other studies define significant fibrosis as F 2 or more. In this study, platelet count (PLT), aspartate aminotransferase (AST), and alkaline phosphatase (ALP) were independent predictors of fibrosis, and PLT, AST, ALP, AST/alanine aminotransferase (ALT) ratio and white blood cell count were independent predictors of cirrhosis.[11] The investigators created models with these variables and concluded that a model with PLT and AST was a simple accurate method to predict advanced fibrosis or cirrhosis. The final model created was termed the APRI, defined as AST (/upper limit of normal [ULN])/PLT (10^9) *100. The area under the receiver operating characteristic curve (AUROC) was used to assess diagnostic accuracy. The AUROC for APRI to predict significant fibrosis was 0.8, and for prediction of cirrhosis, the AUROC was 0.89.[11] Threshold values were identified to predict the absence or presence of significant fibrosis. If APRI was 0.5 or less, significant fibrosis is absent, and if APRI is greater than 1.5, significant fibrosis is present (**Table 2**). In this study, it was estimated that 51% of patients could be accurately predicted to have significant fibrosis or to have absence of significant fibrosis.[11] To

---

Table 1
Additional blood tests and models that have been evaluated to stage liver disease in HCV

Blood Tests	Models
Albumin/total protein[47]	FIBROSpect II[56]
PT[47]	Fibroindex[57]
Immunoglobulins[48]	Hepascore[20]
Insulinlike growth factor 1[49]	SHASTA[58]
α_2-Macroglobulin[50]	Hospital Gregorio Marañón index[59]
Amino-terminal propeptide of type II collagen[26]	Enhanced liver fibrosis test[60]
Matrix metalloproteinase[26]	
Tissue inhibitor of matrix metalloproteinase[51]	
Hyaluronic acid[52]	
High-sensitivity C-reactive protein[52]	
Type IV collagen[53]	
Caspase activity[54]	
Plasma amino acids[55]	
Proteomic markers[50]	
Complement components[50]	

Abbreviation: PT, prothrombin time.

Table 2
Threshold values for assessment of fibrosis biomarkers in the setting of HCV

Test	No Significant Fibrosis (F<2)	Significant Fibrosis (≥F2)
APRI[a]	≤0.5	≥1.5
FibroTest	≤0.1	≥0.6
Forn index	<4.2	>6.9
FIB-4	≤1.45	≥3.25
FibroScan	≤5 kPa	≥7.6 kPa

[a] APRI study defined significant fibrosis as ≥F3.

identify cirrhosis with the APRI, threshold values were identified with APRI of 1.00 or less, indicating absence of cirrhosis and APRI greater than 2 detects cirrhosis. With these threshold values, 81% of patients can be correctly classified as cirrhotic or non-cirrhotic.[11] This model was validated in a validation cohort and by other investigators.[12–14] In a recent meta-analysis of studies assessing the usefulness of APRI in HCV, it was concluded that the APRI was best used to rule out significant fibrosis.[14]

Forns Index

The Forns index was created in a prospective study of patients with hepatitis C undergoing liver biopsy, and a model including demographic variables and laboratory tests was identified to predict presence or absence of fibrosis (stage ≥2 based on the Scheuer classification).[15] The Forns model includes 4 independent predictors of fibrosis, including age, γ-glutamyltransferase (GGT), PLT, and cholesterol level. The Forns index formula is $7.811 - 3.131 \cdot \ln(PLT) + 0.781 \cdot \ln(GGT) + 3.467 \cdot \ln(age) - 0.014 \cdot (cholesterol)$. An AUROC for the Forns index for fibrosis was 0.86 in the test cohort and 0.81 in a validation cohort. Using this model, a cutoff of less than 4.21 was established to predict absence of fibrosis and more than 6.9 significant fibrosis (see **Table 2**). In patients with a score less than 4.21, only 4% had significant fibrosis on the liver biopsy, representing a 96% negative predictive value (NPV). With the application of the Forns index, in patients with a value greater than 6.9, 44% of patients with significant fibrosis in the liver biopsy group were correctly identified; however, this number decreased in the validation cohort. Similar to APRI, the Forns index is more appropriate to use to exclude fibrosis rather than to identify fibrosis.

FIB-4

FIB-4 is a noninvasive marker of fibrosis that was initially developed as a marker of fibrosis in patients with human immunodeficiency virus (HIV)/HCV coinfection.[16] In this retrospective analysis of liver histology and routine blood test results, multivariate logistic regression revealed that age, platelet, and AST were associated with significant fibrosis (Ishak 4–6). These variables were fashioned into a model, termed FIB-4 $(age(year) \times AST (U/L)/(PLT (10^9) \times ALT (U/L))$. Based on this model, one can estimate the degree of liver fibrosis. Using the FIB-4 model, a value of less than 1.45 has an NPV of 90% to exclude advanced fibrosis (Ishak 4–6). For a value greater than 3.25, the FIB-4 had a positive predictive value (PPV) of advanced fibrosis of 65%. Therefore, in most patients with values less than 1.45 or greater than 3.25, a liver biopsy may be avoided[16] (see **Table 2**). Although the FIB-4 was developed in an HIV/HCV-coinfected population, a subsequent study by Vallet-Pichard and colleagues[17] showed that FIB-4 can be applied to HCV-monoinfected patients as well.

FibroTest

Unlike the models that use routine tests, the FibroTest is a noninvasive model that includes several nonroutine tests, including α_2-macroglobulin, apolipoprotein A1, γ-glutamyltranspeptidase, haptoglobin, γ-globulin in addition to total bilirubin. In development of this model, liver biopsies were assessed based on the METAVIR system for substantial fibrosis, F2 or greater, and biopsy specimens were given an activity score (A0–A1 not much activity and A2 or A3 substantial activity), and together with the fibrosis stage, 3 categories were created: (1) without important histologic features (A<2 and F<2), (2) important lesions (A$\geq$2 and F$\geq$2 or both), and (3) widespread fibrosis or cirrhosis (F3 or F4).[18] The AUROC for this model, the FibroTest, was 0.836, and this was replicated in a second group with similar ROC at 0.870. For a score of 0 to 0.1, the NPV was 100% to exclude the presence of significant fibrosis and at scores of 0.60 to 1.00 had a high PPV of more than 90% in identifying the presence of significant fibrosis.[18]

COMPARISONS BETWEEN NONINVASIVE MARKERS OF STAGING FOR HCV

Several studies have compared the performance of noninvasive markers to stage liver disease. In 1 study that compared 9 noninvasive markers, including PLT count, AST/ALT, cirrhosis discriminate score, FIB-4, APRI, age-platelet index (API), Göteborg University cirrhosis index (GUCI), FibroTest, and ActiTest with liver biopsy, FibroTest, FIB-4, APRI, and API all had NPV of greater than 80% to exclude significant fibrosis (compare F0–F2 vs F3–F4)[19] and are better used to exclude significant fibrosis. Vallet-Pichard and colleagues[17] compared FIB-4 and FibroTest in patients with HCV and there was concordance between tests for FIB-4 values less than 1.45 and greater than 3.25. This study showed that FIB-4 can be used in an HCV-monoinfected cohort.[17]

In another study, 9 blood tests (FibroTest, FibroMeter, Forns index, APRI, MP3, the European Liver Fibrosis Group score, Hepascore, FIB-4, and hyaluronate) and TE with FibroScan for liver fibrosis were compared with liver biopsy. FibroScan, FibroMeter, FibroTest, and Hepascore were the optimal tests to detect significant fibrosis and cirrhosis.[20]

In an analysis of 5 study populations, the performance of several markers of fibrosis were assessed including FibroMeter, FibroTest, Hepascore, and APRI. These tests were designed to detect significant fibrosis of F2 or greater.[21] In this study, investigators applied new target end points, including significant fibrosis (F2+F3+F4), severe fibrosis (F3+F4), and cirrhosis (F4). In detection of severe fibrosis, FibroMeter had the highest AUROC, and for cirrhosis, FibroMeter and Hepascore had the highest AUROCs. The AUROCs and accuracies for all tests were higher for cirrhosis than severe fibrosis. This study highlights that the results of blood test or noninvasive marker are dependent on the population studied, the cutoff used, and the diagnostic end point chosen.[21] Therefore, although the absence of fibrosis can be detected with a reasonable degree of accuracy, in patients with test results in the gray zone, further evaluation is required.

FUTURE DEVELOPMENT OF BIOMARKERS FOR FIBROSIS IN HCV

Although the use of biomarkers based on laboratory tests to classify patients with significant fibrosis may reduce the need for liver biopsy, 1 criticism is that these markers are often indeterminate and may not detect those patients with mild to moderate fibrosis or predict those with more rapidly progressive disease.[22] Furthermore, most noninvasive models have similar AUROC values; however, these are compared with the liver biopsy, which, although we consider it a gold standard test to stage liver disease, also has its limitations[23] In addition, because many patients fall in between the upper and lower cutoff values, giving indeterminate results, liver biopsy is still needed in many patients.

Because most of the discussed biomarkers are based on retrospective data to identify biomarkers, including liver function tests as markers of fibrosis, a more accurate assessment of fibrosis based on intermediates or end products of proteins and enzymes involved in the fibrosis pathways may be more accurate. Liver fibrosis involves stellate cell activation and extracellular matrix turnover; therefore, there is interest in development of biomarkers of fibrosis specifically identifying key cytokines and proteins involved in this process. Several biomarkers involved in the fibrosis pathway have already been investigated and include hyaluronic acid, type III procollagen, matrix metalloproteinases, and tissue inhibitors of metalloproteinase.[24–26] Future noninvasive fibrosis tests will likely be based on biomarkers that are functionally related to the pathophysiology of fibrosis development in HCV.[22] These noninvasive markers of fibrosis have also been used to predict histologic progression and clinical outcomes such as hepatic decompensation in patients with HCV cirrhosis.[27]

IMAGING STUDIES

Imaging modalities including magnetic resonance imaging (MRI) and ultrasonography have been studied as noninvasive methods in staging liver disease in the setting of chronic HCV.

ULTRASOUND-BASED MODALITIES
FibroScan

The FibroScan is a portable device that can capture the elasticity of the liver as a marker of fibrosis. The probe has an ultrasound transducer and a vibrator, which is placed in the intercostal space over the right lobe of the liver. A vibration is sent to the tissue to produce a wave that traverses the liver. The ultrasound follows this wave and measures its velocity, which is a measure of tissue stiffness.[28] TE has been studied to determine the degree of fibrosis in liver disease.[29] FibroScan (Echosens, Paris, France) has been studied and compared with liver biopsy results in patients with HCV. The FibroScan probe measures elasticity of the liver, and these results were compared with the activity, steatosis, and fibrosis as assessed on the liver biopsy. There was a high correlation between TE measurements and fibrosis, with a partial correlation coefficient of 0.71 ($P<.001$). In patients with elasticity of 5 kPa or less, 93% had fibrosis stage F0 or F1 and in those with an elasticity of 7.6 kPa or greater, 94% had fibrosis of F2 or greater (see **Table 2**).[29] The FibroScan has limitations in patients with ascites, obesity, or those with narrow intercostal spaces.[29] A prospective study in cirrhotic patients, which assessed factors that negatively affected the performance of FibroScan, found that increased patient age and obesity resulted in lower success rates.[28] Operators who have performed at least 50 previous FibroScan examinations had a higher success rate in capturing shots. It has been suggested that a median of 5 successful measurements with the FibroScan is sufficient to assess for stage of fibrosis in an individual patient.[28]

In addition to FibroScan, acoustic radiation force impulse (ARFI) and supersonic shear imaging (SSI) are ultrasound-based modalities that have been investigated in HCV staging. ARFI uses an ultrasound beam that locally deforms the parenchyma and triggers a shear wave to give a measure of liver stiffness.[30] In a comparison of FibroScan and ARFI with liver biopsy in patients with chronic hepatitis C, the performance of ARFI was superior to FibroScan for diagnosing significant fibrosis ($\geq$F2) and severe fibrosis (F3–F4); however, for cirrhosis, the test performance was equivalent between the 2 modalities.[30] SSI is also an ultrasound-based modality and compared with FibroScan, the SSI technology was more accurate for F2 and greater and F3 and greater; however, they were similar for detecting F = 4 fibrosis.[31] SSI measures a larger area than FibroScan and therefore may be better able to detect fibrosis.[31]

MRI

MRI has been studied in HCV staging with different MRI protocols, including unenhanced MRI, magnetic resonance elastography (MRE), MRI with diffusion-weighted imaging (DWI) and MR spectroscopy. In a study of unenhanced MRI comparing liver biopsy in patients with HCV, although there was a high correlation on MR and certain features of fibrosis and hepatic activity index, the combination of MR features together with laboratory data was superior in detecting inflammation and fibrosis.[32] This study excluded patients with clinical features of portal hypertension, and therefore cannot be applied to patients with cirrhosis.[32] MRI with DWI has been studied and compared with MRE and it has been shown that MRE is superior in predicting fibrosis stage compared with MRI with DWI.[33] MRE has also been compared with ultrasound elastography using FibroScan and APRI for staging liver disease in patients with chronic liver disease.[34] The AUROC for each stage of fibrosis (F>2, F>3, F = 4) was greater for MRE compared with FibroScan, APRI, and FibroScan and APRI together, when comparing accuracy of diagnostic tool with liver biopsy specimens. This study was not performed exclusively in patients with HCV. The benefits of MRE over FibroScan include that this modality can be performed in obese patients and those with ascites.[34] However, MRE is more expensive than FibroScan, which may limit its use.

Breath Tests

Breath tests assess how the liver metabolizes an ingested substance and have been studied as a marker of liver fibrosis in the setting of HCV. The methacetin breath test is based on the fact that ^{13}C-methacetin is metabolized in the liver by cytochrome p450 1A2 into acetaminophen and $^{13}CO_2$ and can therefore be studied as a test of liver function. The methacetin breath test was studied in patients with HCV and control patients.[35] The breath test was able to classify patients as cirrhotic versus noncirrhotic; however, it was unable to differentiate between the various stages of fibrosis.[35] However, by using an algorithm to include breath test parameters, age, and other patient data for both inflammation and fibrosis, in patients with HCV and normal ALT (defined as $\leq$2 ULN), these algorithms were able to differentiate between high and low inflammation and to differentiate between significant and nonsignificant fibrosis in this setting.[36]

An additional breath test that has been studied in HCV is the ^{13}C-aminopyrine breath test. This breath test was able to distinguish control patients from those with chronic hepatitis from patients with Child A cirrhosis early in the breath test.[37] However, at longer time points, there was no difference between patients with hepatitis and cirrhosis. In addition, this breath test was not able to distinguish between high fibrosis scores and cirrhosis.[37] Although breath tests may be able to identify those with cirrhosis at risk for decompensation, they have limited usefulness for accurate assessment of varying degrees of fibrosis.[38]

ALGORITHMS

Several algorithms have been proposed to combine blood tests, models, or FibroScan to improve the accuracy of detecting liver fibrosis and cirrhosis.[39–41]

The SAFE Biopsy

The SAFE (sequential algorithm for fibrosis evaluation) biopsy algorithm has been validated as an algorithm for assessment of fibrosis in HCV.[39] In an international multicenter retrospective study, patients with chronic hepatitis C who underwent liver biopsies also had blood tests for the APRI and FibroTest drawn on the same day. In the SAFE biopsy algorithm, patients have the APRI as an initial screening test, followed by the FibroTest to assess for significant fibrosis of F2 or greater and cirrhosis F4. Application of this algorithm correctly identified most patients, and only 2.6% were misclassified.[39]

Fibropaca Algorithm

The Fibropaca algorithm detects significant fibrosis and cirrhosis based on the use of FibroTest with the APRI and Forns index.[42] With the use of all 3 tests to detect significant fibrosis (F2–F4) and cirrhosis F4, 81.3% of patients were correctly identified comparing their noninvasive markers to liver biopsy.[42] This algorithm suggests performing the FibroTest, the APRI, and Forns index to assess for concordance; if there is no concordance, proceed with a liver biopsy. With this method, 81.3% of patients are correctly identified solely with the combination of noninvasive markers.[42]

Leroy Algorithm

The Leroy algorithm uses APRI and FibroTest simultaneously. This algorithm is useful to detect significant fibrosis (F2–F4) or extensive fibrosis or cirrhosis (F3–F4) using threshold values of FibroTest greater than 0.59 and APRI greater than 2, with a PPV of 96.7% and 92.2%, respectively. The algorithm excluded significant fibrosis (F2–F4) using threshold values of FibroTest less than 0.22 and APRI less than 0.5, with an NPV of 94.1%.[43] This algorithm is useful to discriminate between early and advanced fibrosis. However, there is inadequate information about staging with this algorithm among patients with test values that do not fall within these cutoffs.[43]

In comparing the SAFE biopsy, Fibropaca, and Leroy algorithms, the most accurate algorithm was the Leroy algorithm.[40] However, more biopsies were avoided with Fibropaca, followed by the SAFE biopsy algorithm. The SAFE biopsy and Fibropaca algorithms would be useful in the clinical setting.[40]

IMPLICATIONS OF STAGING VIRAL HEPATITIS C
Treatment Duration

In those with cirrhosis, 48 weeks of treatment with PEG-IFN, ribavirin, and a DAA (boceprevir or telaprevir) is recommended, regardless of virologic response.[44] In contrast, patients without cirrhosis and treatment-naive patients can be treated with response-guided therapy. Therefore, an accurate diagnosis of cirrhosis is imperative in determining treatment duration and counseling about treatment success rates.

Implications of Management

It is imperative not to miss the diagnosis of cirrhosis, because this has important implications. Patients with cirrhosis are at an increased risk of developing HCC and surveillance liver ultrasonography is recommended every 6 months. Patients with cirrhosis are also at risk of developing varices, and these thin-walled veins are at risk of rupture.

An esophagogastroduodenoscopy (EGD) is recommended once a patient is diagnosed with cirrhosis. If the patient develops decompensated cirrhosis, the EGD should be repeated annually.[45] Therefore, it is important to accurately diagnose cirrhosis, because it changes the patient's management and surveillance strategies.

SUMMARY

Accurate assessment of liver fibrosis is essential in the management of those with HCV. It allows identification of those with advanced fibrosis who require periodic surveillance for HCC and esophageal varices. It also identifies those who are not

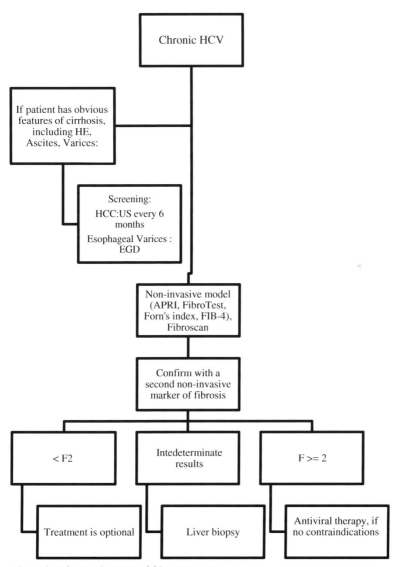

Fig. 1. Algorithm for evaluation of fibrosis in HCV.

candidates for response-guided therapy with DAA. To determine the best option for your patient with chronic HCV requires an understanding of the accuracy and limitations of the models and tests described earlier. We recommend the algorithm depicted in **Fig. 1**.[46] In those with obvious signs of advanced fibrosis (ascites, hepatic encephalopathy, coagulopathy, or significant thrombocytopenia), a biopsy is usually not required. These patients can proceed directly to periodic surveillance for HCC and varices. In those without obvious clinical signs of cirrhosis, we recommend a noninvasive model used alone or in conjunction with a second model for confirmation (ie, APRI, FIB-4, or FibroTest plus FibroScan if available). In those with mild disease (<F2 fibrosis), treatment options include response-guided therapy with DAA combined with PEG-IFN and ribavirin or awaiting interferon-free regimens. Those with fibrosis greater than F2 without cirrhosis are candidates for response-guided therapy, whereas those with cirrhosis are not. Some patients have indeterminate results with noninvasive testing and may still require a liver biopsy. Given the impact that fibrosis has on consequences of chronic HCV and its therapy, accurate staging of fibrosis remains an important aspect in the management of patients with HCV.

REFERENCES

1. Ghany MG, Strader DB, Thomas DL, et al. Diagnosis, management, and treatment of hepatitis C: an update. Hepatology 2009;49:1335–74.
2. Cadranel JF, Rufat P, Degos F. Practices of liver biopsy in France: results of a prospective nationwide survey. For the Group of Epidemiology of the French Association for the Study of the Liver (AFEF). Hepatology 2000;32:477–81.
3. Piccinino F, Sagnelli E, Pasquale G, et al. Complications following percutaneous liver biopsy. A multicentre retrospective study on 68,276 biopsies. J Hepatol 1986;2:165–73.
4. Seeff LB, Everson GT, Morgan TR, et al. Complication rate of percutaneous liver biopsies among persons with advanced chronic liver disease in the HALT-C trial. Clin Gastroenterol Hepatol 2010;8:877–83.
5. Sterling RK, Lyons CD, Stravitz RT, et al. Percutaneous liver biopsy in adult haemophiliacs with hepatitis C virus: safety of outpatient procedure and impact of human immunodeficiency virus coinfection on the spectrum of liver disease. Haemophilia 2007;13:164–71.
6. Sterling RK, Sanyal AJ, Luketic VA, et al. Chronic hepatitis C infection in patients with end stage renal disease: characterization of liver histology and viral load in patients awaiting renal transplantation. Am J Gastroenterol 1999;94:3576–82.
7. Regev A, Berho M, Jeffers LJ, et al. Sampling error and intraobserver variation in liver biopsy in patients with chronic HCV infection. Am J Gastroenterol 2002;97:2614–8.
8. Intraobserver and interobserver variations in liver biopsy interpretation in patients with chronic hepatitis C. The French METAVIR Cooperative Study Group. Hepatology 1994;20:15–20.
9. Schiano TD, Azeem S, Bodian CA, et al. Importance of specimen size in accurate needle liver biopsy evaluation of patients with chronic hepatitis C. Clin Gastroenterol Hepatol 2005;3:930–5.
10. Bedossa P, Dargere D, Paradis V. Sampling variability of liver fibrosis in chronic hepatitis C. Hepatology 2003;38:1449–57.
11. Wai CT, Greenson JK, Fontana RJ, et al. A simple noninvasive index can predict both significant fibrosis and cirrhosis in patients with chronic hepatitis C. Hepatology 2003;38:518–26.

12. Snyder N, Gajula L, Xiao SY, et al. APRI: an easy and validated predictor of hepatic fibrosis in chronic hepatitis C. J Clin Gastroenterol 2006;40:535–42.
13. Al-Mohri H, Cooper C, Murphy T, et al. Validation of a simple model for predicting liver fibrosis in HIV/hepatitis C virus-coinfected patients. HIV Med 2005;6: 375–8.
14. Shaheen AA, Myers RP. Diagnostic accuracy of the aspartate aminotransferase-to-platelet ratio index for the prediction of hepatitis C-related fibrosis: a systematic review. Hepatology 2007;46:912–21.
15. Forns X, Ampurdanes S, Llovet JM, et al. Identification of chronic hepatitis C patients without hepatic fibrosis by a simple predictive model. Hepatology 2002;36:986–92.
16. Sterling RK, Lissen E, Clumeck N, et al. Development of a simple noninvasive index to predict significant fibrosis in patients with HIV/HCV coinfection. Hepatology 2006;43:1317–25.
17. Vallet-Pichard A, Mallet V, Nalpas B, et al. FIB-4: an inexpensive and accurate marker of fibrosis in HCV infection. Comparison with liver biopsy and fibrotest. Hepatology 2007;46:32–6.
18. Imbert-Bismut F, Ratziu V, Pieroni L, et al. Biochemical markers of liver fibrosis in patients with hepatitis C virus infection: a prospective study. Lancet 2001;357: 1069–75.
19. Usluer G, Erben N, Aykin N, et al. Comparison of non-invasive fibrosis markers and classical liver biopsy in chronic hepatitis C. Eur J Clin Microbiol Infect Dis 2012;31(8):1873–8.
20. Zarski JP, Sturm N, Guechot J, et al. Comparison of nine blood tests and transient elastography for liver fibrosis in chronic hepatitis C: the ANRS HCEP-23 study. J Hepatol 2012;56:55–62.
21. Boursier J, Bacq Y, Halfon P, et al. Improved diagnostic accuracy of blood tests for severe fibrosis and cirrhosis in chronic hepatitis C. Eur J Gastroenterol Hepatol 2009;21:28–38.
22. Martinez SM, Crespo G, Navasa M, et al. Noninvasive assessment of liver fibrosis. Hepatology 2011;53:325–35.
23. Mehta SH, Lau B, Afdhal NH, et al. Exceeding the limits of liver histology markers. J Hepatol 2009;50:36–41.
24. Rosenberg WM, Voelker M, Thiel R, et al. Serum markers detect the presence of liver fibrosis: a cohort study. Gastroenterology 2004;127:1704–13.
25. Fontana RJ, Goodman ZD, Dienstag JL, et al. Relationship of serum fibrosis markers with liver fibrosis stage and collagen content in patients with advanced chronic hepatitis C. Hepatology 2008;47:789–98.
26. Leroy V, Monier F, Bottari S, et al. Circulating matrix metalloproteinases 1, 2, 9 and their inhibitors TIMP-1 and TIMP-2 as serum markers of liver fibrosis in patients with chronic hepatitis C: comparison with PIIINP and hyaluronic acid. Am J Gastroenterol 2004;99:271–9.
27. Fontana RJ, Dienstag JL, Bonkovsky HL, et al. Serum fibrosis markers are associated with liver disease progression in non-responder patients with chronic hepatitis C. Gut 2010;59:1401–9.
28. Kettaneh A, Marcellin P, Douvin C, et al. Features associated with success rate and performance of FibroScan measurements for the diagnosis of cirrhosis in HCV patients: a prospective study of 935 patients. J Hepatol 2007;46:628–34.
29. Sandrin L, Fourquet B, Hasquenoph JM, et al. Transient elastography: a new noninvasive method for assessment of hepatic fibrosis. Ultrasound Med Biol 2003;29:1705–13.

30. Rizzo L, Calvaruso V, Cacopardo B, et al. Comparison of transient elastography and acoustic radiation force impulse for non-invasive staging of liver fibrosis in patients with chronic hepatitis C. Am J Gastroenterol 2011;106:2112–20.

31. Bavu E, Gennisson JL, Couade M, et al. Noninvasive in vivo liver fibrosis evaluation using supersonic shear imaging: a clinical study on 113 hepatitis C virus patients. Ultrasound Med Biol 2011;37:1361–73.

32. Mitchell DG, Navarro VJ, Herrine SK, et al. Compensated hepatitis C: unenhanced MR imaging correlated with pathologic grading and staging. Abdom Imaging 2008;33:58–64.

33. Wang Y, Ganger DR, Levitsky J, et al. Assessment of chronic hepatitis and fibrosis: comparison of MR elastography and diffusion-weighted imaging. AJR Am J Roentgenol 2011;196:553–61.

34. Huwart L, Sempoux C, Vicaut E, et al. Magnetic resonance elastography for the noninvasive staging of liver fibrosis. Gastroenterology 2008;135:32–40.

35. Braden B, Faust D, Sarrazin U, et al. 13C-methacetin breath test as liver function test in patients with chronic hepatitis C virus infection. Aliment Pharmacol Ther 2005;21:179–85.

36. Lalazar G, Pappo O, Hershcovici T, et al. A continuous 13C methacetin breath test for noninvasive assessment of intrahepatic inflammation and fibrosis in patients with chronic HCV infection and normal ALT. J Viral Hepat 2008;15:716–28.

37. Giannini E, Fasoli A, Chiarbonello B, et al. 13C-aminopyrine breath test to evaluate severity of disease in patients with chronic hepatitis C virus infection. Aliment Pharmacol Ther 2002;16:717–25.

38. Everson GT, Shiffman ML, Hoefs JC, et al. Quantitative liver function tests improve the prediction of clinical outcomes in chronic hepatitis C: results from the Hepatitis C Antiviral Long-Term Treatment Against Cirrhosis Trial. Hepatology 2012;55:1019–29.

39. Sebastiani G, Halfon P, Castera L, et al. SAFE biopsy: a validated method for large-scale staging of liver fibrosis in chronic hepatitis C. Hepatology 2009;49:1821–7.

40. Sebastiani G, Halfon P, Castera L, et al. Comparison of three algorithms of noninvasive markers of fibrosis in chronic hepatitis C. Aliment Pharmacol Ther 2012;35:92–104.

41. Castera L, Sebastiani G, Le Bail B, et al. Prospective comparison of two algorithms combining non-invasive methods for staging liver fibrosis in chronic hepatitis C. J Hepatol 2010;52:191–8.

42. Bourliere M, Penaranda G, Renou C, et al. Validation and comparison of indexes for fibrosis and cirrhosis prediction in chronic hepatitis C patients: proposal for a pragmatic approach classification without liver biopsies. J Viral Hepat 2006;13:659–70.

43. Leroy V, Hilleret MN, Sturm N, et al. Prospective comparison of six non-invasive scores for the diagnosis of liver fibrosis in chronic hepatitis C. J Hepatol 2007;46:775–82.

44. Ghany MG, Nelson DR, Strader DB, et al. An update on treatment of genotype 1 chronic hepatitis C virus infection: 2011 practice guideline by the American Association for the Study of Liver Diseases. Hepatology 2011;54:1433–44.

45. Garcia-Tsao G, Sanyal AJ, Grace ND, et al. Prevention and management of gastroesophageal varices and variceal hemorrhage in cirrhosis. Hepatology 2007;46:922–38.

46. Smith JO, Sterling RK. Systematic review: non-invasive methods of fibrosis analysis in chronic hepatitis C. Aliment Pharmacol Ther 2009;30:557–76.

47. Benlloch S, Heredia L, Barquero C, et al. Prospective validation of a noninvasive index for predicting liver fibrosis in hepatitis C virus-infected liver transplant recipients. Liver Transpl 2009;15:1798–807.
48. Watt K, Uhanova J, Gong Y, et al. Serum immunoglobulins predict the extent of hepatic fibrosis in patients with chronic hepatitis C virus infection. J Viral Hepat 2004;11:251–6.
49. Lorenzo-Zuniga V, Bartoli R, Masnou H, et al. Serum concentrations of insulin-like growth factor-I (igf-I) as a marker of liver fibrosis in patients with chronic hepatitis C. Dig Dis Sci 2007;52:3245–50.
50. Gangadharan B, Antrobus R, Dwek RA, et al. Novel serum biomarker candidates for liver fibrosis in hepatitis C patients. Clin Chem 2007;53:1792–9.
51. Larrousse M, Laguno M, Segarra M, et al. Noninvasive diagnosis of hepatic fibrosis in HIV/HCV-coinfected patients. J Acquir Immune Defic Syndr 2007;46: 304–11.
52. Yilmaz S, Bayan K, Tuzun Y, et al. Replacement of histological findings: serum hyaluronic acid for fibrosis, high-sensitive C-reactive protein for necroinflammation in chronic viral hepatitis. Int J Clin Pract 2007;61:438–43.
53. Murawaki Y, Koda M, Okamoto K, et al. Diagnostic value of serum type IV collagen test in comparison with platelet count for predicting the fibrotic stage in patients with chronic hepatitis C. J Gastroenterol Hepatol 2001;16:777–81.
54. Bantel H, Lugering A, Poremba C, et al. Caspase activation correlates with the degree of inflammatory liver injury in chronic hepatitis C virus infection. Hepatology 2001;34:758–67.
55. Zhang Q, Takahashi M, Noguchi Y, et al. Plasma amino acid profiles applied for diagnosis of advanced liver fibrosis in patients with chronic hepatitis C infection. Hepatol Res 2006;34:170–7.
56. Zaman A, Rosen HR, Ingram K, et al. Assessment of FIBROSpect II to detect hepatic fibrosis in chronic hepatitis C patients. Am J Med 2007;120(280):e9–14.
57. Koda M, Matunaga Y, Kawakami M, et al. FibroIndex, a practical index for predicting significant fibrosis in patients with chronic hepatitis C. Hepatology 2007;45:297–306.
58. Kelleher TB, Mehta SH, Bhaskar R, et al. Prediction of hepatic fibrosis in HIV/HCV co-infected patients using serum fibrosis markers: the SHASTA index. J Hepatol 2005;43:78–84.
59. Berenguer J, Bellon JM, Miralles P, et al. Identification of liver fibrosis in HIV/HCV-coinfected patients using a simple predictive model based on routine laboratory data. J Viral Hepat 2007;14:859–69.
60. Parkes J, Guha IN, Roderick P, et al. Enhanced Liver Fibrosis (ELF) test accurately identifies liver fibrosis in patients with chronic hepatitis C. J Viral Hepat 2011;18:23–31.

IL28B Polymorphisms as a Pretreatment Predictor of Response to HCV Treatment

Christoph T. Berger, MD[a,b,c], Arthur Y. Kim, MD[d],*

KEYWORDS

- IL28B • Pharmacogenomics • Antiviral • Type III interferon • Interferon-lambda

KEY POINTS

- Polymorphisms related to the gene encoding IL28B are the strongest genetic predictors of HCV clearance, both by interferon-based treatment or by the natural immune system.
- IL28B belongs to the interferon-lambda family and plays a plausible biologic role in antiviral defenses.
- The predictive capacity of IL28B is thus far strongest for HCV genotypes 1 and 4.
- The effects of IL28B extend into special populations with HCV, such as those with HIV-1 coinfection and liver transplant recipients.
- IL28B polymorphisms will continue to play a role as a clinical pharmacogenomic test in the current direct-acting antiviral era and may be relevant as interferon-free regimens are developed.

INTRODUCTION

Approximately 170 million individuals, or about 2% to 3% of the world's population, are chronically infected with the hepatitis C virus (HCV).[1] With the approval of interferon (IFN) alfa for HCV treatment in 1991, infection could be successfully cured in only a fraction of patients. The first combination treatment with ribavirin (RBV) and replacement of conventional IFN with pegylated IFN alfa (PEG-IFNa) led to dramatically increased treatment success rates during the past decade. Still, about half of all affected individuals fail to clear the virus despite this treatment.[2] Several viral and host factors (infection with HCV genotype 1 and 4, higher magnitude of viral titers,

[a] Ragon Institute of Massachusetts General Hospital, Massachusetts Institute of Technology and Harvard Medical School, Boston, MA 02129, USA; [b] Department of Internal Medicine, University Hospital Basel, Basel, Switzerland; [c] Department of Biomedicine, University Hospital Basel, Basel, Switzerland; [d] Division of Infectious Diseases, Massachusetts General Hospital, Harvard Medical School, 55 Fruit Street, Cox 5, Boston, MA 02114, USA
* Corresponding author.
E-mail address: akim1@partners.org

Infect Dis Clin N Am 26 (2012) 863–877
http://dx.doi.org/10.1016/j.idc.2012.08.010
0891-5520/12/$ – see front matter © 2012 Elsevier Inc. All rights reserved.

id.theclinics.com

male gender, advanced liver fibrosis, and African ancestry) were associated with poor treatment response rates.[3] Stratification based on such risk factors consequently led to personalized treatment strategies that varied mostly in the duration of treatment.[2] Because PEG-IFNa/RBV is hampered by its long duration and the high burden of side effects, even more accurate predictors of outcome would help clinicians optimize treatment plans and duration.

This motivated several genome-wide association studies (GWAS) aimed at identifying protective host genetic factors associated with successful treatment response or spontaneous HCV clearance. In 2009 and 2010 several groups independently reported single nucleotide polymorphisms (SNP) near the interleukin-28β subunit (IL28B) gene that were dramatically associated with sustained virologic response (SVR) to PEG-IFNa/RBV and spontaneous viral clearance in the absence of therapy.[4–7] IL28B genotyping quickly became available in research and clinical settings and a large number of studies investigating the impact of the IL28B genotype have been published since the first reports. Just as these discoveries heralded a new era in HCV treatment based on pharmacogenomic testing, several questions remain regarding the use of IL28B genotype testing in clinical practice.

GWAS TO DETECT HOST GENETIC FACTORS IN HCV IDENTIFIES AN SNP LINKING IL28B TO TREATMENT RESPONSE

The human genome spans more than 3 billion base pairs with an overall conservation rate of more than 99%. GWAS test a set of more than 500,000 SNPs that commonly occur in a population (eg, >5%), and SNP frequencies are compared between a cohort of individuals with a specific condition or disease outcome and respective controls.[8] Importantly, in most cases the SNPs that are detected are not contained within the genes involved in the different outcome, but rather are often upstream or downstream and therefore are "tags" of the genes themselves. Thus, after an SNP is detected, a subsequent fine mapping of the area of interest is warranted. Moreover, because several SNPs in that area can tag the same gene, testing for "linkage disequilibrium" (the degree these SNPs are linked on the same chromosome) is crucial. Overall, a genome-wide approach's major advantage is that associations can be screened for in an unbiased and hypothesis-free manner, contrary to studies where target genes are specifically selected and thus by design prevents the discovery of new and unexpected genetic associations.

The first independent GWAS were performed in patients receiving PEG-IFNa/RBV for genotype 1 HCV infection and discovered two SNPs (rs12979860 and rs 8099917) on chromosome 19, which were located in close proximity to the IL28B gene, a type III IFN with antiviral and immunomodulatory effects.[4–7] These were some of the strongest associations identified in any GWAS to date.[9] In the first study, being homozygous for the favorable SNP of rs12979860 (C/C genotype), depending on the ethnic background, resulted in an odds ratio of 5.6 to 7.3 compared with the C/T or T/T genotype to achieve SVR. This favorable effect was strongest in whites, but was found to be independent of gender, ethnicity, liver fibrosis, or pretreatment viral loads. The beneficial SNP was much more common in whites compared with individuals of African descent, and accounted for roughly 50% of the difference in the treatment response between these two groups.[4] Interestingly, homozygosity for the favorable allele of rs12979860 was also associated with natural or "spontaneous" clearance of infection, suggesting shared mechanisms of viral control between both types of clearance.[10] These host genotypes do not influence control of other chronic viruses, such as HIV-1 or hepatitis B virus.[11,12]

Subsequently, three additional GWAS conducted in Australian, Japanese, and Swiss HCV cohorts identified another SNP, rs8099917, in the IL28B genomic region that was significantly associated with treatment response.[5–7] Importantly, this SNP is in strong linkage with rs12979860 and was the second strongest SNP identified in the study by Ge and colleagues[4] before correcting for rs12979860. Furthermore, rs12979860 was not or only partially assessed in the other GWAS, thus explaining why top hits differed.[13]

Several lines of evidence indicate that the IL28B gene is the causative gene for the difference in viral clearance: (1) the IL28B gene lies in close proximity to both identified SNPs (rs12979860 and rs8099917); (2) subsequent fine mapping of the IL28B gene region identified two SNP of potential importance in linkage disequilibrium with the previously mentioned SNPs, one of them a nonsynonymous change in the gene (rs8103142) resulting in a lysine to arginine substitution at position 70 (K70R), and another SNP (rs28416813) only 37 base pairs upstream of the IL28B translation initiation site[7,14]; (3) the favorable IL28B genotype associates with increased IL28B levels, suggesting a functional importance of the protein[15]; and (4) previous studies indicated similar functional proprieties of type III IFN and type I IFN,[16] providing biologic plausibility that IL28B may be beneficial in HCV clearance. This immediate plausibility contrasts with genetic associations found by GWAS for other diseases, where the links to pathogenesis are often not immediately obvious.

BIOLOGY, FUNCTION, AND CLINICAL APPLICATION OF TYPE III IFN IN CLINICAL TRIALS

IL28B is a cytokine of the type III IFN family, with IL28A and IL29 being the other members. Several cell types are capable of expressing IL28B in response to viral infections. Dendritic cells and macrophages, and primary hepatocytes and hepatic tumor lines, have been shown to produce IL28B after contact with HCV.[17–20] IL28B signals through a heterodimeric receptor composed of one part IL-28Rα (also called IL-28R1) and one part IL-10R2.[21,22] The IL-28Rα is expressed at high levels on hepatocytes, suggesting that IL28B is involved in antiviral activity in the infected liver.[17,23,24] In fact, type III IFNs inhibit HCV replication in vitro comparable with type I IFN.[25,26] Other cell types, including B lymphocytes and T lymphocytes, have been reported to express this receptor at varying levels and thus additional immunomodulatory functions compared with type I IFN are likely.[23,24] However, exactly how and to what extent, IL28B directly contributes to HCV clearance in vivo remains poorly understood. IL28B shares several functional characteristics with type I IFN, including antiviral activity and immunomodulatory function.[21,22,27,28]

The strong genetic link between IL28B genotype and HCV clearance, alongside the strong IL28B production seen in natural HCV infection in primates,[29] supports the idea that IL28B might be a potential treatment for HCV infection.[16] Currently, there are no data available from IL28B trials. However, preliminary results from clinical trials with another type III IFN, IL29, structurally and functionally very similar to IL28B, show early promise as effective antiviral therapy. In 86% of the treatment-naive patients who received combined PEG IL29 and RBV for 4 weeks there was a relevant decrease in HCV viral load observed.[30] Intriguingly, compared with PEG-IFNa treatment, it seems that many of the adverse effects seen with PEG-IFNa therapy are not induced by type III IFN, likely explained by the restricted expression of IFN-lambda receptors to certain cell types compared with those of IFN-alfa, which are expressed on virtually all cell types.[30] Phase II trials comparing IL29 and PEG-IFNa are currently ongoing (Genzyme/Bristol Myers, clinical trials.gov).

IL28B HOMOZYGOSITY FOR THE FAVORABLE ALLELE IS LINKED TO RAPID VIROLOGIC RESPONSE

Despite this strong evidence for an important role of IL28B in HCV treatment response, the phenotype that explains the different outcomes remains largely unknown. One study looked at the viral suppression in the first 24 hours after treatment initiation and found that the favorable genotype was highly predictive of rapid decline of viremia.[31] In line with this, rapid virologic response (RVR) rate was significantly higher in individuals with the favorable genotype.[32] This could mechanistically be explained by studies looking at the gene expression profiles in HCV, suggesting that the favorable genotype has lower pretreatment interferon-stimulated gene expression, a state that predicts response rate to IFNa treatment even better than the IL28B genotype alone.[33] However, individuals with RVR had the highest rate of SVR, independent of the host IL28B genotype, suggesting that other (IL28B independent) mechanisms may help to achieve a positive outcome in some individuals with nonfavorable IL28B genotypes.

PREDICTIVE VALUE OF IL28B GENOTYPE IN NON–GENOTYPE 1 INFECTION

The first GWAS on factors predicting HCV SVR focused on those with genotype 1, the most common genotype in the developed world. Determining the influence of IL28B host polymorphisms on non–genotype 1 outcomes was the next logical extension of these findings, because treatment of genotype 1 with PEG-IFNa/RBV has much lower SVR rates (40%–45%) than genotype 2 or 3 (65%–82%).[3,34] This was addressed in a large randomized, controlled trial in 268 individuals infected with HCV genotype 2/3 that compared treatment with PEG-IFNa/RBV for 24 weeks (SOC group) with 12 weeks if they had a RVR or with 24 weeks if they did not achieve RVR (response-guided group). In this setting the favorable IL28B allele was only associated with SVR in individuals without RVR in the SOC group but did not affect RVR in either group.[35] Similarly, Moghaddam and colleagues[36] found no impact of the IL28B genotype on SVR in a cohort of 281 individuals infected with genotype 3 (except between the C/C and T/T carriers); however, having both favorable alleles of IL28B was associated with RVR in this study, a finding confirmed by others.[36,37] Several other studies supported a lack of association of IL28B genotype with SVR in genotype 2/3 infection,[38–40] including a large Asian study focusing on genotype 2 only.[40] Conversely, others reported that the favorable allele predicts SVR (particularly after failure to achieve RVR) in genotype 2/3 infection[41] and that a beneficial effect of the favorable IL28B allele on SVR might be strongest in genotype 2b.[38,42] The lower rates of nonresponse in genotype 2/3 infection may have reduced power to detect significant differences. Taken together, data suggest that any beneficial effect of the favorable IL28B genotype for genotype 2/3 would be at lower strength compared with genotype 1 infection.

In Western countries HCV genotype 4 is rare, but represents the most common genotype in some areas including Egypt, which has one of the highest HCV prevalence worldwide. Previously, several small studies that included individuals infected with genotype 4 consistently reported effects of the IL28B genotype comparable with those seen in genotype 1 HCV infection.[5,43,44] These findings were recently confirmed in two larger trials including 112 and 82 individuals infected with genotype 4, respectively.[45,46] In one study by De Nicola and colleagues[45] homozygote carriers of the good IL28B allele had an SVR rate of 88% compared with 38%, and showed no relapses (vs 36% in the CT/TT group). Asselah and colleagues[46] found similar associations with clearance rates of 81.8% in the CC carriers versus 46.5% and 29.4% in the CT and TT carriers, respectively.

Finally, genotype 5 is most prevalent in South Africa or Syria, but clusters have also been reported in Spain, Belgium, and France. Because of its relative rarity, genotype 5 is often neglected in clinical trials. In 49 infected individuals of white descent, there were no differences in the SVR rate by IL28B genotype.[47] Whether this lack of association is caused by small sample size or by the older age and higher fibrosis grade in these individuals infected with genotype 5 remains elusive.

In summary, IL28B genotype strongly predicts treatment response in HCV genotype 1 and 4 infection, may or may not predict response in genotype 2 and 3, and more data are needed to determine prediction of response in genotype 5. Thus, it is recommended that IL28B testing only be performed for genotype 1 and 4 infections.

PREDICTIVE VALUE OF IL28B IN SPECIAL POPULATIONS AND POTENTIAL USE IN LIVER TRANSPLANTATION FOR HCV

IL28B SNPs and their influence in viral clearance was first discovered in patients who were monoinfected with HCV alone. Subsequently, the finding was rapidly extended to specialized populations, such as those with coexisting HIV-1 infection.[5,44,48–51] In perinatal studies, no association was found with the rate of HCV transmission but the same host genotypes are associated with spontaneous clearance in children.[52]

In the posttransplant setting for HCV, infection of the newly placed graft is virtually universal and cases of spontaneous clearance are extraordinarily rare; because of their rarity IL28B genotypes have yet to be linked to this outcome. For IFN-based treatment outcomes in the posttransplant setting, several studies show that if either the donor or recipient IL28B genotype was favorable, SVR rates were improved, but even more so when both donor and recipient were favorable.[53–56] These studies suggest that the mechanisms by which IL28B genotypes influence treatment response are more likely to be related to innate responses than adaptive responses, given the significant defects in the latter induced by exogenous immunosuppression posttransplant. Moreover, they suggest the possibility of allocating liver grafts based on favorable donor IL28B genotype to those with HCV to enhance the likelihood of response to IFN-based therapies. Further information is required before such allocation can be implemented, including the role of IL28B in the rapid fibrosis progression observed in the posttransplant setting. IL28B genotypes favorable for treatment response could lead to better viral control or slower progression or to more brisk inflammation and rapid progression. Thus far early posttransplant studies suggest that recipient alleles unfavorable for treatment response are associated with more rapid progression[53,57] but that the opposite may hold for the donor IL28B genotypes.[58] Whether patients homozygous for the favorable allele experience more rapid fibrosis progression in the nontransplant setting remains an open question.[59]

USE OF HOST IL28B GENOTYPING FOR ACUTE GENOTYPE 1 INFECTION

Because IL28B genotype is also a strong predictor of spontaneous resolution of HCV in genotype 1 infection,[10] there may be a role for testing in the setting of acute infection when the outcome is yet to be determined. In particular testing may help select individuals that would profit most from immediate treatment (IL28B genotypes suggesting progression to chronic infection) or that would be given a chance to be observed to see if spontaneous clearance occurs, thus saving treatment (IL28B favorable genotype). Interestingly, favorable genotype was associated with symptoms during acute HCV, which is also a predictor of spontaneous clearance.[60,61] Patients might initially defer treatment knowing that spontaneous clearance rates might be as high as 64% with CC rs12979860 genotype[61] and initiate only if serial viral titers suggest that the patient will not clear. By contrast, the low spontaneous clearance rate in individuals with the unfavorable IL28B genotype (24% in the heterozygote CT and 6% in the homozygote TT) is a strong argument to treat these individuals as early as possible, especially if not symptomatic.[61,62] The counterargument to testing in the acute setting is that IL28B is an imperfect predictor of spontaneous clearance; up to 36% of the individuals with the favorable genotype will not clear infection and that treatment response to PEG-IFNa–based regimens is generally higher if started in acute HCV infection. Finally, IL28B does not predict SVR when PEG-IFNa is applied in the acute phase and thus has diminished use.[60]

A recent model-based analysis contradicted such IL28B-guided approaches, showing that immediate treatment of all acutely infected individuals (independent of IL28B genotype and presence of HCV related symptoms) may be the best approach to reduce the development of chronic HCV roughly by half.[63] The currently available data therefore suggest that IL28B genotype in acute HCV infection should not be used as a sole argument to withhold early treatment in individuals with the favorable genotype,[2] but could rather be used in conjunction with other predictors of clearance (**Box 1**, **Table 1**) to help clinicians and patients to weigh the individual chance of spontaneous resolution against potential treatment-associated side effects. Finally, although generating predictive models is informative[64] clearly prospective studies are needed to inform evidence-based recommendations.

USE OF HOST IL28B GENOTYPING FOR CHRONIC GENOTYPE 1 INFECTION IN THE DIRECT-ACTING ANTIVIRAL ERA

Recently, several trials of new direct acting antivirals (DAA) have generated exciting results with increased SVR in treatment-naive subjects and relapsers (for recent reviews on the topic see[73,74]). Intriguingly, preliminary data suggest that these agents might be successful even in IFN-free treatment regimens.[75] These drugs will revolutionize HCV treatment and combination treatments promise effective treatments of previously refractory HCV infection in the near future. Data from available studies on DAAs indicate an increased SVR rate independent of the IL28B genotype, but specifically individuals infected with HCV with the unfavorable IL28B genotypes showed the largest increase in SVR when a DAA was added to the treatment.[76,77] Thus, one might argue that DAAs should be part of every HCV treatment strategy in the future for genotype 1 and thus the discovery of the IL28B genotype came a little too late.[78,79]

However, it is more likely that IL28B plays a role even in the current DAA era (with IFN) and beyond. There remain several potential applications of IL28B testing to individualize treatments in specific HCV patient subgroups. Because of the differences in treatment outcome depending on the viral genotype and other individual factors (see **Table 1**), clinicians treating HCV-infected individuals are experienced in using such genetic predictors and biomarkers to select the appropriate RBV dose and treatment length. The reproducible and strong association of favorable HCV outcome in various clinical settings with the good IL28B allele, and relatively easy testing and broad availability of the test, holds promise for its applicability in clinical decision-making.

The most obvious application of IL28B genotype testing could be to identify subjects who might profit the most of the addition of a protease inhibitor to PEG-IFNa/RBV. A potential approach could be to immediately add a protease inhibitor to PEG-IFNa/RBV in patients with a nonfavorable IL28B genotype, whereas treat those with favorable IL28B genotypes initially with PEG-IFNa/RBV alone. For individuals with the good IL28B genotype DAAs could be made available as add-on treatment for those not achieving initial RVR.[80] Because protease inhibitor treatment is

Table 1
Viral and host factors predicting treatment response to interferon-based regimens in hepatitis C virus

Predictor of Better Treatment Response	References
Viral	
Rapid virologic response (negative viral load at Week 4 on therapy)[a]	3
Hepatitis C virus genotype 2/3	3,64
Low baseline viremia	3,64
Female gender	3,87
Viral polymorphisms (ie, baseline predominating resistance mutations)	88
Genotype 1b vs 1a	88,89
Host	
Demographic	
Normal body mass index	90
Younger age	64,87
White or East Asian ethnicity	3,91,92
Adherence to antiviral medications	93,94
Serum markers	
Low inducible protein-10 levels	95,96
Cytokine levels	87
High vitamin D_3 levels	97,98
Intrahepatic factors	
Absence or low liver fibrosis	3
Low pretreatment hepatic ISG expression[a]	33,99
High RIG1/ISG15	100
Factors in immune cells	
Myxovirus-resistance protein A gene expression in macrophages	101
Genetic factors	
IL28B genotype[a]	4–7
Killer-immunoglobulin–like receptor genotype	102–104
Human leukocyte antigen DQB1	105
Programmed death-1 polymorphism	106

Abbreviations: ISG, interferon-stimulated genes; RIG-1, retinoic acid-inducible gene I.
[a] Factors associated with IL28B genotyping, others are independent.

expensive (about \$1100–\$4300 per week, depending on the agent) such an approach would reduce overall costs.[81]

Optimizing the treatment duration has been one of the hot topics in HCV research. Although genotype 1 infection is usually treated for 48 weeks, those with RVR can be reduced to 24 weeks.[2,82] Similarly, although a 24-week duration of therapy is used in genotype 2 and 3 infection, the length of treatment can be shortened to 12 to 16 weeks if RVR is achieved.[2,83] Not surprisingly, the IL28B genotype has been shown to affect RVR in two large trials of boceprevir/PEG-IFNa/RBV (RESPOND-2/SPRINT-2) and thus might be used to predict if shorter treatment duration is an option.[84,85] A counter-argument is that because RVR is the stronger predictor of SVR than IL28B, genotyping may not change clinical practice; in other words, success during the initial period of therapy trumps the genetic predictor and can render it unnecessary. Similarly, retrospective analysis of individuals with the favorable genotype that did not achieve

> **Box 1**
> **Arguments or potential applications for and against IL28B testing in the clinical setting**
>
> *Pro IL28B genotype testing*
>
> - Allows pretreatment prediction of response to PEG-IFNa[4–7]
> - Shorter treatment might be an option in non-GT1 infected with the favorable IL28B genotype[65–67]
> - Treatment intensification in non-RVR with nonfavorable IL28B GT[35]
> - Adding a direct-acting antivirals to PEG-IFNa/RBV in GT1-infected individuals with the nonfavorable IL28B genotype[2]
> - Shorter triple therapies in the presence of the favorable IL28B genotype[68,69]
> - Longer treatment (72 weeks) of GT1/4 in slow responders increases SVR rate[70]
> - Consider retreatment of GT1 infection with treatment failure and the favorable IL28B genotype[71]
>
> *Against IL28B genotype testing*
>
> - Viral kinetics (especially RVR) are better predictors of SVR than the IL28B genotype[3] (ie, in non-RVR with the good genotype treatment probably cannot be shortened[72])
> - Not enough data to withhold direct-acting antivirals in the favorable IL28B genotype[2]
> - Negative predictive value is too low to really chose not to treat based on the expected SVR[6]
> - In the near future everybody will receive triple therapy because SVR might be up to 100% after only 12 weeks of triple therapy in the good IL28B genotype[68]

RVR showed no evidence that in these patients shorter treatment duration of 24 weeks would suffice.[72]

A few studies have also looked at whether IL28B genotype can be used to intensify treatment dose or duration. In fact, a higher dose of PEG-IFNa resulted in higher response rate in individuals with previous treatment failure heterozygous for the IL28B allele versus those homozygous for the bad allele.[86] For individuals infected with genotype 2 or 3 current standard of care is a 24-week treatment course of PEG-IFNa/RBV and addition of the currently available DAAs is not necessary because of high efficacy in their absence (genotype 2) and lack of predicted activity (genotype 3). Nonetheless, IL-28B testing may predict whether certain individuals with the nonfavorable host genotype should consider treatment extension from the usual 24 to 48 weeks.[35] Similarly, in genotype 1 and 4 infection treatment extension to 72 weeks in nonresponders or slow responders with the nonfavorable IL28B genotype might increase SVR substantially to PEG-IFNa/RBV alone (13% vs 61%), although this strategy is likely unpalatable in the DAA era.[70] However, it is likely that this might be different in the setting of triple therapy including a DAA, where 12 weeks of treatment resulted in 100% SVR in individuals with the good genotype versus 40% and 20% in heterozygote or homozygote bad allele carriers.[68]

SUMMARY

Pretreatment determination of IL28B genotype in patients chronically infected with genotype 1 may assist the decision process by supplying the provider and patient some insight into the expected outcome on so-called triple therapy. A host IL28B genotype may affect a decision regarding whether a specific patient should be treated or not with current available therapies: a more favorable genotype may favor an initially less intensive approach with PEG-IFNa/RBV and using viral kinetics to guide use of an additional protease inhibitor. In contrast, a less favorable genotype may require a more aggressive approach upfront or even consideration of deferral until even newer treatment paradigms are available. For patients already motivated or in need of therapy, early viral kinetics remain better predictors than IL28B and thus testing may not change the decision to treat; however, testing may still affect duration of therapy. Because data from prospective and randomized trials are lacking to date, most of these applications remain speculative and their use requires confirmation.

The role of IL28B in the future era of IFN-free regimens remains to be determined. A key component of future studies using IFN-free strategies will be close study of those with unsuccessful treatment because of nonresponse or relapse and whether the mechanisms of IL28B will influence these results. Because of the fundamental role of IL28B as a predictor of HCV clearance, the initial reports of relapse while on IFN-free therapy,[75] and the possibility of using IFN-based strategies as salvage for IFN-free ones, testing for IL28B polymorphisms is likely to retain relevance even as therapeutic paradigms evolve.

REFERENCES

1. Alter MJ. Epidemiology of hepatitis C virus infection. World J Gastroenterol 2007;13(17):2436–41.
2. Ghany MG, Nelson DR, Strader DB, et al. An update on treatment of genotype 1 chronic hepatitis C virus infection: 2011 practice guideline by the American Association for the Study of Liver Diseases. Hepatology 2011;54(4):1433–44.
3. McHutchison JG, Lawitz EJ, Shiffman ML, et al. Peginterferon alfa-2b or alfa-2a with ribavirin for treatment of hepatitis C infection. N Engl J Med 2009;361(6):580–93.
4. Ge D, Fellay J, Thompson AJ, et al. Genetic variation in IL28B predicts hepatitis C treatment-induced viral clearance. Nature 2009;461(7262):399–401.
5. Rauch A, Kutalik Z, Descombes P, et al. Genetic variation in IL28B is associated with chronic hepatitis C and treatment failure: a genome-wide association study. Gastroenterology 2010;138(4):1338–45, 1345.e1–7.
6. Suppiah V, Moldovan M, Ahlenstiel G, et al. IL28B is associated with response to chronic hepatitis C interferon-alpha and ribavirin therapy. Nat Genet 2009; 41(10):1100–4.
7. Tanaka Y, Nishida N, Sugiyama M, et al. Genome-wide association of IL28B with response to pegylated interferon-alpha and ribavirin therapy for chronic hepatitis C. Nat Genet 2009;41(10):1105–9.
8. Pearson TA, Manolio TA. How to interpret a genome-wide association study. JAMA 2008;299(11):1335–44.
9. Hindorff L, MacArthur J, Wise A, et al. A catalog of published genome-wide association studies. Available at: http://www.genome.gov/gwastudies. Accessed September 29, 2012.
10. Thomas DL, Thio CL, Martin MP, et al. Genetic variation in IL28B and spontaneous clearance of hepatitis C virus. Nature 2009;461(7265):798–801.
11. Martin MP, Qi Y, Goedert JJ, et al. IL28B polymorphism does not determine outcomes of hepatitis B virus or HIV infection. J Infect Dis 2010;202(11): 1749–53.
12. Salgado M, Kirk GD, Cox A, et al. Protective interleukin-28B genotype affects hepatitis C virus clearance, but does not contribute to HIV-1 control in a cohort of African-American elite controllers/suppressors. AIDS 2011;25(3):385–7.
13. Balagopal A, Thomas DL, Thio CL. IL28B and the control of hepatitis C virus infection. Gastroenterology 2010;139(6):1865–76.

14. de Castellarnau M, Aparicio E, Parera M, et al. Deciphering the interleukin 28B variants that better predict response to pegylated interferon-alpha and ribavirin therapy in HCV/HIV-1 coinfected patients. PLoS One 2012;7(2):e31016.

15. Langhans B, Kupfer B, Braunschweiger I, et al. Interferon-lambda serum levels in hepatitis C. J Hepatol 2011;54(5):859–65.

16. Donnelly RP, Dickensheets H, O'Brien TR. Interferon-lambda and therapy for chronic hepatitis C virus infection. Trends Immunol 2011;32(9):443–50.

17. Pagliaccetti NE, Robek MD. Interferon-λ in the immune response to hepatitis B virus and hepatitis C virus. J Interferon Cytokine Res 2010;30(8):585–90.

18. Coccia EM, Severa M, Giacomini E, et al. Viral infection and Toll-like receptor agonists induce a differential expression of type I and λ interferons in human plasmacytoid and monocyte-derived dendritic cells. Eur J Immunol 2004; 34(3):796–805.

19. Megjugorac NJ, Gallagher GE, Gallagher G. IL-4 enhances IFN-{lambda}1 (IL-29) production by plasmacytoid DCs via monocyte secretion of IL-1Ra. Blood 2010;115(21):4185–90.

20. Mihm S, Frese M, Meier V, et al. Interferon type I gene expression in chronic hepatitis C. Lab Invest 2004;84(9):1148–59.

21. Kotenko SV, Gallagher G, Baurin VV, et al. IFN-[lambda]s mediate antiviral protection through a distinct class II cytokine receptor complex. Nat Immunol 2003;4(1):69–77.

22. Sheppard P, Kindsvogel W, Xu W, et al. IL-28, IL-29 and their class II cytokine receptor IL-28R. Nat Immunol 2003;4(1):63–8.

23. Witte K, Gruetz G, Volk HD, et al. Despite IFN-[lambda] receptor expression, blood immune cells, but not keratinocytes or melanocytes, have an impaired response to type III interferons: implications for therapeutic applications of these cytokines. Genes Immun 2009;10(8):702–14.

24. Doyle SE, Schreckhise H, Khuu-Duong K, et al. Interleukin-29 uses a type 1 interferon-like program to promote antiviral responses in human hepatocytes. Hepatology 2006;44(4):896–906.

25. Marcello T, Grakoui A, Barba-Spaeth G, et al. Interferons alpha and lambda inhibit hepatitis C virus replication with distinct signal transduction and gene regulation kinetics. Gastroenterology 2006;131(6):1887–98.

26. Robek MD, Boyd BS, Chisari FV. Lambda interferon inhibits hepatitis B and C virus replication. J Virol 2005;79(6):3851–4.

27. O'Brien TR. Interferon-alfa, interferon-lambda and hepatitis C. Nat Genet 2009; 41(10):1048–50.

28. Zhang L, Jilg N, Shao RX, et al. IL28B inhibits hepatitis C virus replication through the JAK-STAT pathway. J Hepatol 2011;55(2):289–98.

29. Thomas E, Gonzalez VD, Li Q, et al. HCV infection induces a unique hepatic innate immune response associated with robust production of type III interferons. Gastroenterology 2012;142(4):978–88.

30. Muir AJ, Shiffman ML, Zaman A, et al. Phase 1b study of pegylated interferon lambda 1 with or without ribavirin in patients with chronic genotype 1 hepatitis C virus infection. Hepatology 2010;52(3):822–32.

31. Bochud PY, Bibert S, Negro F, et al. IL28B polymorphisms predict reduction of HCV RNA from the first day of therapy in chronic hepatitis C. J Hepatol 2011; 55(5):980–8.

32. Thompson AJ, Muir AJ, Sulkowski MS, et al. Interleukin-28B polymorphism improves viral kinetics and is the strongest pretreatment predictor of sustained

virologic response in genotype 1 hepatitis C virus. Gastroenterology 2010; 139(1):120–129.e18.

33. Dill MT, Duong FH, Vogt JE, et al. Interferon-induced gene expression is a stronger predictor of treatment response than IL28B genotype in patients with hepatitis C. Gastroenterology 2011;140(3):1021–31.

34. Manns MP, McHutchison JG, Gordon SC, et al. Peginterferon alfa-2b plus ribavirin compared with interferon alfa-2b plus ribavirin for initial treatment of chronic hepatitis C: a randomised trial. Lancet 2001;358(9286):958–65.

35. Mangia A, Thompson AJ, Santoro R, et al. An IL28B polymorphism determines treatment response of hepatitis C virus genotype 2 or 3 patients who do not achieve a rapid virologic response. Gastroenterology 2010;139(3):821–7, 827.e1.

36. Moghaddam A, Melum E, Reinton N, et al. IL28B genetic variation and treatment response in patients with hepatitis C virus genotype 3 infection. Hepatology 2011;53(3):746–54.

37. Lindh M, Lagging M, Farkkila M, et al. Interleukin 28B gene variation at rs12979860 determines early viral kinetics during treatment in patients carrying genotypes 2 or 3 of hepatitis C virus. J Infect Dis 2011;203(12):1748–52.

38. Kawaoka T, Hayes CN, Ohishi W, et al. Predictive value of the IL28B polymorphism on the effect of interferon therapy in chronic hepatitis C patients with genotypes 2a and 2b. J Hepatol 2011;54(3):408–14.

39. Scherzer TM, Hofer H, Staettermayer AF, et al. Early virologic response and IL28B polymorphisms in patients with chronic hepatitis C genotype 3 treated with peginterferon alfa-2a and ribavirin. J Hepatol 2011;54(5):866–71.

40. Yu ML, Huang CF, Huang JF, et al. Role of interleukin-28B polymorphisms in the treatment of hepatitis C virus genotype 2 infection in Asian patients. Hepatology 2011;53(1):7–13.

41. Sarrazin C, Susser S, Doehring A, et al. Importance of IL28B gene polymorphisms in hepatitis C virus genotype 2 and 3 infected patients. J Hepatol 2011;54(3):415–21.

42. Sakamoto N, Nakagawa M, Tanaka Y, et al. Association of IL28B variants with response to pegylated-interferon alpha plus ribavirin combination therapy reveals intersubgenotypic differences between genotypes 2a and 2b. J Med Virol 2011;83(5):871–8.

43. Stattermayer AF, Stauber R, Hofer H, et al. Impact of IL28B genotype on the early and sustained virologic response in treatment-naive patients with chronic hepatitis C. Clin Gastroenterol Hepatol 2011;9(4):344–350.e2.

44. Rallon NI, Naggie S, Benito JM, et al. Association of a single nucleotide polymorphism near the interleukin-28B gene with response to hepatitis C therapy in HIV/hepatitis C virus-coinfected patients. AIDS 2010;24(8):F23–9.

45. De Nicola S, Aghemo A, Rumi MG, et al. Interleukin 28B polymorphism predicts pegylated interferon plus ribavirin treatment outcome in chronic hepatitis C genotype 4. Hepatology 2012;55(2):336–42.

46. Asselah T, De Muynck S, Broet P, et al. IL28B polymorphism is associated with treatment response in patients with genotype 4 chronic hepatitis C. J Hepatol 2012;56(3):527–32.

47. Antaki N, Bibert S, Kebbewar K, et al. IL28B polymorphisms do not predict response to therapy in chronic hepatitis C with HCV genotype 5. Gut 2012;61: 1640–1.

48. Pineda JA, Caruz A, Rivero A, et al. Prediction of response to pegylated interferon plus ribavirin by IL28B gene variation in patients coinfected with HIV and hepatitis C virus. Clin Infect Dis 2010;51(7):788–95.

49. Dayyeh BK, Gupta N, Sherman KE, et al. IL28B alleles exert an additive dose effect when applied to HCV-HIV coinfected persons undergoing peginterferon and ribavirin therapy. PLoS One 2011;6(10):e25753.

50. Labarga P, Barreiro P, Mira JA, et al. Impact of IL28B polymorphisms on response to peginterferon and ribavirin in HIV-hepatitis C virus-coinfected patients with prior nonresponse or relapse. AIDS 2011;25(8):1131–3.

51. Neukam K, Camacho A, Caruz A, et al. Prediction of response to pegylated interferon plus ribavirin in HIV/hepatitis C virus (HCV)-coinfected patients using HCV genotype, IL28B variations, and HCV-RNA load. J Hepatol 2012;56(4):788–94.

52. Ruiz-Extremera A, Munoz-Gamez JA, Salmeron-Ruiz MA, et al. Genetic variation in interleukin 28B with respect to vertical transmission of hepatitis C virus and spontaneous clearance in HCV-infected children. Hepatology 2011;53(6):1830–8.

53. Charlton MR, Thompson A, Veldt BJ, et al. Interleukin-28B polymorphisms are associated with histological recurrence and treatment response following liver transplantation in patients with hepatitis C virus infection. Hepatology 2011;53(1):317–24.

54. Coto-Llerena M, Perez-Del-Pulgar S, Crespo G, et al. Donor and recipient IL28B polymorphisms in HCV-infected patients undergoing antiviral therapy before and after liver transplantation. Am J Transplant 2011;11(5):1051–7.

55. Fukuhara T, Taketomi A, Motomura T, et al. Variants in IL28B in liver recipients and donors correlate with response to peg-interferon and ribavirin therapy for recurrent hepatitis C. Gastroenterology 2010;139(5):1577–85, 1585.e1–3.

56. Lange CM, Moradpour D, Doehring A, et al. Impact of donor and recipient IL28B rs12979860 genotypes on hepatitis C virus liver graft reinfection. J Hepatol 2011;55(2):322–7.

57. Graziadei IW, Zoller HM, Schloegl A, et al. Early viral load and recipient interleukin-28B rs12979860 genotype are predictors of the progression of hepatitis C after liver transplantation. Liver Transpl 2012;18(6):671–9.

58. Duarte-Rojo A, Veldt BJ, Goldstein DD, et al. The course of posttransplant hepatitis C infection: comparative impact of donor and recipient source of the favorable IL28B genotype and other variables. Transplantation 2012;94(2):197–203.

59. Barreiro P, Pineda JA, Rallon N, et al. Influence of interleukin-28B single-nucleotide polymorphisms on progression to liver cirrhosis in human immunodeficiency virus-hepatitis C virus-coinfected patients receiving antiretroviral therapy. J Infect Dis 2011;203(11):1629–36.

60. Grebely J, Petoumenos K, Hellard M, et al. Potential role for interleukin-28B genotype in treatment decision-making in recent hepatitis C virus infection. Hepatology 2010;52(4):1216–24.

61. Tillmann HL, Thompson AJ, Patel K, et al. A polymorphism near IL28B is associated with spontaneous clearance of acute hepatitis C virus and jaundice. Gastroenterology 2010;139(5):1586–92, 1592.e1.

62. Grebely J, Matthews GV, Dore GJ. Treatment of acute HCV infection. Nat Rev Gastroenterol Hepatol 2011;8(5):265–74.

63. Deuffic-Burban S, Castel H, Wiegand J, et al. Immediate vs. delayed treatment in patients with acute hepatitis C based on IL28B polymorphism: a model-based analysis. J Hepatol 2012;57(2):260–6.

64. Ochi H, Hayes CN, Abe H, et al. Toward the establishment of a prediction system for the personalized treatment of chronic hepatitis C. J Infect Dis 2012;205(2):204–10.

65. Liu CH, Liang CC, Liu CJ, et al. Interleukin 28B genetic polymorphisms and viral factors help identify HCV genotype-1 patients who benefit from 24-week pegylated interferon plus ribavirin therapy. Antivir Ther 2012;17(3):477–84.
66. Rallon NI, Soriano V, Naggie S, et al. IL28B gene polymorphisms and viral kinetics in HIV/hepatitis C virus-coinfected patients treated with pegylated interferon and ribavirin. AIDS 2011;25(8):1025–33.
67. Scherzer TM, Stattermayer AF, Strasser M, et al. Impact of IL28B on treatment outcome in hepatitis C virus G1/4 patients receiving response-guided therapy with peginterferon alpha-2a (40KD)/ribavirin. Hepatology 2011;54(5):1518–26.
68. Bronowicki J, Hezode C, Bengtsson L, et al. 100% SVR in IL28B SNP rs12979860 C/C patients treated with 12 weeks of telaprevir, peginterferon and ribavirin in the PROVE2 trial EASL 2012. Barcelona (Spain); 2012.
69. McHutchison JG, Manns MP, Muir AJ, et al. Telaprevir for previously treated chronic HCV infection. N Engl J Med 2010;362(14):1292–303.
70. Pearlman BL, Ehleben C. The IL-28B genotype predicts which slow-responding hepatitis C-infected patients will benefit from treatment extension. Am J Gastroenterol 2011;106(7):1370–1.
71. O'Bryan JM, Potts JA, Bonkovsky HL, et al. Extended interferon-alpha therapy accelerates telomere length loss in human peripheral blood T lymphocytes. PLoS One 2011;6(8):e20922.
72. Huang CF, Huang JF, Yang JF, et al. Interleukin-28B genetic variants in identification of hepatitis C virus genotype 1 patients responding to 24 weeks peginterferon/ribavirin. J Hepatol 2012;56(1):34–40.
73. Barritt ASIV, Fried MW. Maximizing opportunities and avoiding mistakes in triple therapy for hepatitis C virus. Gastroenterology 2012;142(6):1314–1323.e1.
74. Welsch C, Jesudian A, Zeuzem S, et al. New direct-acting antiviral agents for the treatment of hepatitis C virus infection and perspectives. Gut 2012;61(Suppl 1): i36–46.
75. Lok AS, Gardiner DF, Lawitz E, et al. Preliminary study of two antiviral agents for hepatitis C genotype 1. N Engl J Med 2012;366(3):216–24.
76. Jacobson IM, McHutchison JG, Dusheiko G, et al. Telaprevir for previously untreated chronic hepatitis C virus infection. N Engl J Med 2011;364(25):2405–16.
77. Poordad F, McCone J Jr, Bacon BR, et al. Boceprevir for untreated chronic HCV genotype 1 infection. N Engl J Med 2011;364(13):1195–206.
78. Hofmann WP, Zeuzem S. A new standard of care for the treatment of chronic HCV infection. Nat Rev Gastroenterol Hepatol 2011;8(5):257–64.
79. Jensen DM, Pol S. IL28B genetic polymorphism testing in the era of direct acting antivirals therapy for chronic hepatitis C: ten years too late? Liver Int 2012; 32(Suppl 1):74–8.
80. Fried M, Buti M, Dore G. Efficacy and safety of TMC435 in combination with pegintereron alfa 2a and ribavirin in treatment-naïve genotype-1 HCV patients: 24-week interim results from the PILLAR study. Hepatology 2010;52(Suppl 4): LB-5.
81. Liu S, Cipriano LE, Holodniy M, et al. New protease inhibitors for the treatment of chronic hepatitis C: a cost-effectiveness analysis. Ann Intern Med 2012;156(4): 279–90.
82. Moreno C, Deltenre P, Pawlotsky JM, et al. Shortened treatment duration in treatment-naive genotype 1 HCV patients with rapid virological response: a meta-analysis. J Hepatol 2010;52:25–31.
83. European Association for the Study of the Liver. EASL clinical practice guidelines: management of hepatitis C virus infection. J Hepatol 2011;55(2):245–64.

84. Zeuzem S, Asselah T, Angus P, et al. Efficacy of the protease inhibitor BI 201335, polymerase inhibitor BI 207127, and ribavirin in patients with chronic HCV infection. Gastroenterology 2011;141(6):2047–55 [quiz: e14].

85. Bacon BR, Gordon SC, Lawitz E, et al. Boceprevir for previously treated chronic HCV genotype 1 infection. N Engl J Med 2011;364(13):1207–17.

86. Chevaliez S, Hezode C, Soulier A, et al. High-dose pegylated interferon-alpha and ribavirin in nonresponder hepatitis C patients and relationship with IL-28B genotype (SYREN trial). Gastroenterology 2011;141(1):119–27.

87. Gao B, Hong F, Radaeva S. Host factors and failure of interferon-alpha treatment in hepatitis C virus. Hepatology 2004;39(4):880–90.

88. Lim SR, Qin X, Susser S, et al. Virologic escape during danoprevir (ITMN-191/RG7227) monotherapy is hepatitis C virus subtype dependent and associated with R155 K substitution. Antimicrob Agents Chemother 2012;56(1):271–9.

89. Vispo E, Rallon NI, Labarga P, et al. Different impact of IL28B polymorphisms on response to peginterferon-alpha plus ribavirin in HIV-positive patients infected with HCV subtypes 1a or 1b. J Clin Virol 2012;55(1):58–61.

90. Walsh MJ, Jonsson JR, Richardson MM, et al. Non-response to antiviral therapy is associated with obesity and increased hepatic expression of suppressor of cytokine signalling 3 (SOCS-3) in patients with chronic hepatitis C, viral genotype 1. Gut 2006;55(4):529–35.

91. Muir AJ, Bornstein JD, Killenberg PG. Peginterferon alfa-2b and ribavirin for the treatment of chronic hepatitis C in blacks and non-Hispanic whites. N Engl J Med 2004;350(22):2265–71.

92. Dev AT, McCaw R, Sundararajan V, et al. Southeast Asian patients with chronic hepatitis C: the impact of novel genotypes and race on treatment outcome. Hepatology 2002;36(5):1259–65.

93. Lo Re VIII, Teal V, Localio AR, et al. Relationship between adherence to hepatitis C virus therapy and virologic outcomes: a cohort study. Ann Intern Med 2011;155(6):353–60.

94. Lo Re VIII, Amorosa VK, Localio AR, et al. Adherence to hepatitis C virus therapy and early virologic outcomes. Clin Infect Dis 2009;48(2):186–93.

95. Romero AI, Lagging M, Westin J, et al. Interferon (IFN)-gamma-inducible protein-10: association with histological results, viral kinetics, and outcome during treatment with pegylated IFN-alpha 2a and ribavirin for chronic hepatitis C virus infection. J Infect Dis 2006;194(7):895–903.

96. Casrouge A, Decalf J, Ahloulay M, et al. Evidence for an antagonist form of the chemokine CXCL10 in patients chronically infected with HCV. J Clin Invest 2011;121(1):308–17.

97. Petta S, Camma C, Scazzone C, et al. Low vitamin D serum level is related to severe fibrosis and low responsiveness to interferon-based therapy in genotype 1 chronic hepatitis C. Hepatology 2010;51(4):1158–67.

98. Bitetto D, Fattovich G, Fabris C, et al. Complementary role of vitamin D deficiency and the interleukin-28B rs12979860 C/T polymorphism in predicting antiviral response in chronic hepatitis C. Hepatology 2011;53(4):1118–26.

99. Honda M, Sakai A, Yamashita T, et al. Hepatic ISG expression is associated with genetic variation in interleukin 28B and the outcome of IFN therapy for chronic hepatitis C. Gastroenterology 2010;139(2):499–509.

100. Asahina Y, Tsuchiya K, Muraoka M, et al. Association of gene expression involving innate immunity and genetic variation in interleukin 28B with antiviral response. Hepatology 2012;55(1):20–9.

101. McGilvray I, Feld JJ, Chen L, et al. Hepatic cell-type specific gene expression better predicts HCV treatment outcome than IL28B genotype. Gastroenterology 2012;142(5):1122–1131.e1.

102. Khakoo SI, Thio CL, Martin MP, et al. HLA and NK cell inhibitory receptor genes in resolving hepatitis C virus infection. Science 2004;305(5685):872–4.

103. Dring MM, Morrison MH, McSharry BP, et al. Innate immune genes synergize to predict increased risk of chronic disease in hepatitis C virus infection. Proc Natl Acad Sci U S A 2011;108(14):5736–41.

104. Suppiah V, Gaudieri S, Armstrong NJ, et al. IL28B, HLA-C, and KIR variants additively predict response to therapy in chronic hepatitis C virus infection in a European Cohort: a cross-sectional study. PLoS Med 2011;8(9):e1001092.

105. de Rueda PM, Lopez-Nevot MA, Saenz-Lopez P, et al. Importance of host genetic factors HLA and IL28B as predictors of response to pegylated interferon and ribavirin. Am J Gastroenterol 2011;106(7):1246–54.

106. Vidal-Castineira JR, Lopez-Vazquez A, Alonso-Arias R, et al. A predictive model of treatment outcome in patients with chronic HCV infection using IL28B and PD-1 genotyping. J Hepatol 2012;56(6):1230–8.

The Importance of Rapid Viral Suppression in the Era of Directly Acting Antiviral Therapy for Hepatitis C Virus

Erin T. Jenkins, MD[a],*, Donald M. Jensen, MD[b]

KEYWORDS

- Hepatitis C • Direct-acting antiviral agents • Boceprevir • Telaprevir
- Rapid viral response • Extended rapid viral response

KEY POINTS

- Rapid viral response (undetectable viral load at week 4) is a strong predictor of eventual sustained viral response to therapy with pegylated interferon and ribavirin, and triple therapy with protease inhibitors.
- Therapy with direct-acting antiviral agents results in rapid decrease in viral load.
- Resistant viral variants develop quickly in patients who do not experience rapid or sustained viral clearance.
- Many patients with rapid and extended viral clearance are eligible for shortened 24-week courses of triple therapy.
- Patients with slow virologic response are unlikely to benefit from further therapy and may be eligible for early termination of therapy.

BACKGROUND

Although non-A, non-B hepatitis was recognized as a major cause of parenteral post-transfusion hepatitis beginning in the 1970s, hepatitis C virus (HCV) was not isolated as the causative agent until 1989.[1] Initial trials investigating interferon therapy for treatment of HCV monitored liver chemistry tests and biopsy specimens to measure response to therapy, because serum HCV polymerase chain reaction (PCR) tests were not yet available.[2–4] However, using liver enzymes to measure response to

[a] Section of Gastroenterology, Hepatology, and Nutrition, University of Chicago Medical Center, MC 4076 Room M 421, 5841 South Maryland, Chicago, IL 60637, USA; [b] Center for Liver Diseases, University of Chicago Medical Center, 5841 South Maryland, MC7120, Chicago, IL 60637, USA
* Corresponding author.
E-mail address: Erin.Jenkins@uchospitals.edu

Infect Dis Clin N Am 26 (2012) 879–891
http://dx.doi.org/10.1016/j.idc.2012.08.007
0891-5520/12/$ – see front matter © 2012 Published by Elsevier Inc.

id.theclinics.com

therapy has its limitations, because changes in enzymes do not always correlate with changes in viral activity,[5] and may be influenced by a direct or immune-mediated effect of interferon.[6] The discovery and refinement of a quantitative HCV PCR assay to measure viral load in the early 1990s allowed for an advanced understanding of the virus and treatment.

LESSONS FROM HIV

An understanding of viral kinetics was noted to be critical in clinical HIV therapy, and lessons learned in HIV treatment influenced understanding of HCV therapy. Researchers found that the HIV virus replicates rapidly, with frequent errors that produce new variants, some with drug resistance even in patients who were never exposed to antiretroviral medications.[7] In the early treatment era, use of monotherapy led to the rapid emergence of these resistant minority species. In contrast, plasma HIV RNA levels decrease rapidly in patients on effective combination drug regimens comprising a minimum of 2 drug classes. While on potent antiretroviral therapy, most patients achieve undetectable levels within 2 to 3 months of effective therapy. However, incomplete viral suppression in some patients allows for the rapid accumulation of new mutations, including possible drug-resistant variants. This event underscores the importance of early, complete viral suppression.[7]

VIRAL KINETICS AS A MEASUREMENT OF RESPONSE

The measurement of HCV RNA viral load changes during interferon therapy was first described in 1991. A retrospective analysis of serum from patients in one of the early interferon trials noted that most of the biochemical responders had decreased levels of HCV RNA during treatment, and many of those with sustained normalization of aminotransferases also had sustained undetectable HCV RNA.[8] Retrospective and prospective studies confirmed that pretreatment viral load and viral genotype and fibrosis score all independently predicted response to standard interferon therapy.[9,10] More recently, a host genetic polymorphism on chromosome 19, *IL28B*, was shown to be the most impactful pretherapy predictor of response.[11]

EARLY VIRAL KINETICS WITH INTERFERON AND RIBAVIRIN

Early studies of viral kinetics in the setting of interferon monotherapy showed a biphasic response. The first phase consists of a rapid, exponential, dose-dependent decline of virus within 24 hours. In the second phase, decline is slower and variable among patients.[12] The rate of second-phase decline is influenced by interferon effectiveness and loss of infected hepatocytes.[12] Although important in preventing therapeutic relapse after discontinuation of combination therapy, ribavirin alone has minimal effect on viral kinetics.[13] However, some have speculated that the "shoulder" observed between the first and second phases of interferon/ribavirin combination therapy may represent a unique ribavirin effect on viral mutagenesis or possibly an increase in immune clearance.[14]

VIRAL KINETICS AND STANDARD INTERFERON-BASED THERAPY

Early experience with interferon monotherapy showed that 85% of the biochemical response occurred in the first 3 months, and that ongoing treatment was unlikely to cause further decrease in liver enzymes. Based on this knowledge, the 1997 National Institutes of Health consensus guidelines recommended stopping therapy in those who do not experience normalization of aminotransferases by 3 months, because of the low probability of any further benefit.[15] Studies using hepatitis V viral load confirmed the importance of early viral decline in predicting eventual sustained response. A prospective trial of interferon monotherapy found that half of the patients who were HCV RNA–undetectable by 48 hours were still undetectable at 6 months, and none of those with positive HCV RNA at 48 hours were undetectable by 6 months.[16] None of the patients with positive HCV RNA at week 8 were undetectable at the end of the trial.[10] The stopping rule was then modified to reflect the availability of viral assays, and anyone with either persistent aminotransferase elevation or persistent detectable virus at 12 weeks on interferon monotherapy was allowed to stop treatment.

Combination therapy with interferon and ribavirin was confirmed to be superior to interferon monotherapy, increasing sustained virologic response (SVR) rate from 13% (48 weeks of interferon monotherapy) to 38% (48 weeks of interferon plus ribavirin).[17] A large prospective trial of interferon with ribavirin combination therapy showed that half of the patients who had persistent viremia at week 12 of combination therapy eventually attained a sustained viral response.[17] Treatment guidelines were then readjusted to allow a minimum of 24 weeks of dual therapy for all patients regardless of viral levels at week 12 (**Table 1**).

EARLY VIROLOGIC RESPONSE

Researchers examined viral kinetics more closely to better predict response to combination therapy. Two retrospective reviews of multicenter trials of PegIFN with ribavirin therapy found that failure to decrease viral load by 2 logs by the 12th week of therapy, defined as the early virologic response (EVR), was a strong predictor of nonresponse. Only 0% to 3% of patients who did not achieve EVR would experience SVR.[18,19] Patients who attained a 2-log decline in viral load by week 12 but had persistent virus had viral levels rechecked at week 24. Those who reached EVR at week 12 but retained a detectable virus at week 24 had only a 4% chance of attaining SVR.[18] Current guidelines support stopping therapy with PegIFN and ribavirin at 12 weeks in anyone who fails to achieve EVR.[20] Despite the near 100% negative predictive value of failure to achieve EVR, this same benchmark is not a strong positive predictor of SVR, with only 65% to 72% of those experiencing EVR attaining SVR on combination therapy.[18,19,21] However, a complete EVR, defined as undetectable HCV RNA at week 12, was found to be a better predictor of sustained response, and 75% to 84% of patients with HCV of mixed genotypes with complete EVR at 12 weeks ultimately attained SVR with interferon-based therapy (**Table 2**).[18]

Table 1	
Virologic response during therapy and definitions	
Response	**Definition**
RVR Rapid virologic response	HCV RNA–negative at 4 wk as defined by HCV RNA <50 IU/mL
EVR Early virologic response	HCV RNA–negative or $\geq 2 \log_{10}$ drop at wk 12
Relapse	HCV RNA–negative at end of treatment but HCV RNA positive after treatment cessation
SVR Sustained virologic response	HCV RNA–negative 24 wk after end of treatment

Table 2	
Virologic response at week 12 and definitions	
EVR Early virologic response	HCV RNA–negative or $\geq 2 \log_{10}$ decrease at wk 12
Complete EVR	No RVR but HCV RNA–negative (<50 IU/mL) at wk 12
Partial EVR	No RVR and detectable but $\geq 2 \log_{10}$ decrease in HCV RNA at wk 12
○ Slow responder	$\geq 2 \log_{10}$ decrease in HCV RNA at wk 12 and HCV RNA–negative at wk 4
○ Partial responder	$\geq 2 \log_{10}$ decrease in HCV RNA at wk 12 but HCV RNA–positive at wk 24

RAPID VIRAL RESPONSE IN GENOTYPE 1: PREDICTOR OF SVR

Rapid viral response (RVR) is defined as an undetectable HCV RNA level by treatment week 4, and has been found to be a strong predictor of SVR.[21,22] RVR has a positive predictive value of SVR of 87.5% in genotype 1, whereas the negative predictive value is only 56.1% to 74%.[21,22] Thus, although a positive RVR is highly predictive of response, a negative RVR should not be used as an indication to stop therapy. Those with RVR have such a favorable response to therapy and low rates of relapse that many can achieve SVR with only 24 weeks of dual therapy. Unfortunately, fewer than one-quarter of patients with genotype 1 on dual therapy achieve RVR. A post hoc analysis of a large prospective trial comparing 24-and 48-week regimens of PegIFN with varying dosing of ribavirin showed an overall RVR rate of approximately 24% in those with genotype 1.[23,24] Of those who obtained RVR, 89% in the 24-week treatment group achieved SVR, which was similar to the response in the 48-week group.[24] A prospective study comparing patients with genotype 1 chronic hepatitis C (CHC) with low pretreatment viral loads undergoing 24 weeks of PegIFN versus historical controls receiving 48 weeks of therapy confirmed that, in those with RVR, 24 weeks of therapy produced similar SVR rates (89% and 85%, respectively) as 48 weeks of therapy (**Fig. 1**).[25]

EARLY NULL RESPONSE

Earlier predictors of poor response are beneficial, identifying patients unlikely to respond and allowing them to discontinue therapy earlier to avoid unnecessary cost

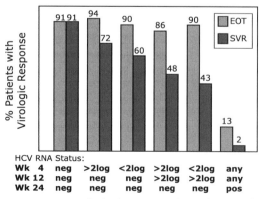

Fig. 1. SVR rates by on-treatment virologic response in patients undergoing PegIFN and ribavirin therapy. (*Courtesy of* Dr Donald Jensen, Chicago, IL).

and potential side effects. Early null response (ENR) is defined as failure to achieve a 1-log decline in viral load by week 4 on therapy. A retrospective study examining patients on combination PegIFN/ribavirin therapy showed that ENR has a high negative predictive value. Of the patients in the cohort, 24% were null responders and only 8% of these experienced SVR.[26] ENR had a 92% negative predictive value for SVR and, as a predictor of non response, would misclassify only 2% of all patients in the entire cohort. ENR identified 68% of all patients who would not achieve EVR, and has been proposed as a possible new stopping point for standard therapy.

DIRECT-ACTING ANTIVIRAL AGENTS

An increased understanding of viral kinetics has allowed clinicians to tailor HCV therapy to patients, identifying those who have the best chance of viral eradication and those who will likely fail therapy. Nonetheless, SVR rates with PegIFN and ribavirin remain disappointingly low, with SVR rates around 40% to 50% for patients with genotype 1, and even lower in patients with unfavorable *IL28B* genotypes. However, exciting advancements in hepatitis C therapy include the development of new direct-acting antiviral (DAA) agents that offer much higher rates of sustained viral eradication when used in combination with PegIFN and ribavirin. Two orally available protease inhibitors specific for NS3/4a serine protease have been approved for use in the treatment of genotype 1 chronic hepatitis C—boceprevir (Victrelis) and telaprevir (Incivek)—and many other agents are under investigation. Rapid viral suppression is key in the efficacy of these drugs, and all clinical trials with these agents have incorporated measurement of viral kinetics.

VIRAL KINETICS WITH DAA MONOTHERAPY
DAA Monotherapy

Single-agent DAA therapy with either boceprevir or telaprevir results in a rapid decrease in viral load, but the response is not sustained, with frequent breakthrough and relapse.[27,28] Virus replicates rapidly but with frequent errors, allowing for the selection of resistant variants. This experience mirrors with single-drug therapy in HIV, and prompted trials of combination therapy using DAA agents combined with PegIFN and ribavirin.

Triple Therapy

Clinical trials of telaprevir
The first, small, phase 1 study investigating telaprevir triple therapy assigned 12 patients with genotype 1 HCV to receive telaprevir with PegIFN/ribavirin for 4 weeks, with the option for patients to continue PegIFN/ribavirin therapy for 44 additional weeks.[29] All patients were treatment-naïve, and those with cirrhosis or hepatitis B or HIV coinfections were excluded. Viral clearance with triple therapy was rapid, and 2 patients had undetectable HCV RNA by day 8; 100% experienced RVR. No breakthrough occurred during triple therapy, and many patients who continued therapy with PegIFN/ribavirin ultimately attained SVR, including one patient who discontinued therapy at week 22.[29]

PROVE1, a phase 2b multicenter, randomized, double-blind trial, investigated the efficacy of 12 weeks of telaprevir combined with 12, 24, or 48 weeks of PegIFN/ribavirin for HCV genotype 1 compared with 48 weeks of PegIFN/ribavirin alone.[30] All arms including telaprevir had a higher proportion of patients achieving rapid viral clearance than the control group; 81% of patients receiving telaprevir and 24 to 48 weeks of PegIFN/ribavirin achieved RVR, compared with only 11% of the control group. SVR was significantly higher in the groups receiving 12 weeks of telaprevir with 24 weeks of PegIFN/ribavirin (61%) and receiving 12 weeks of telaprevir with 48 weeks of PegIFN/ribavirin (67%) compared with controls (41%). Viral breakthrough was uncommon, occurring in 7% of patients in telaprevir-based groups. Most viral breakthroughs occurred early, by week 4, and all breakthroughs occurred within 12 weeks. Telaprevir-resistant mutations were seen in most patients who experienced break-through. Most of those with resistant variants (10/12) were genotype 1a subtype, because this subtype has a lower barrier to the formation of resistant variants.[30] This study proved that adding telaprevir to standard therapy increased rates of SVR, and suggested that it may be possible to shorten treatment duration to 24 weeks.

PROVE2 trial

This phase 2b multicentre, randomized, partially double-blind, placebo-controlled trial investigated the efficacy of telaprevir with PegIFN with or without ribavirin for varying lengths of treatment.[31] The mean time to viral clearance was 22 to 29 days in the telaprevir-containing groups compared with 113 days in the PegIFN/ribavirin group. Viral breakthrough was very common in patients receiving telaprevir and PegIFN without ribavirin; patients assigned to this treatment arm also had a lower SVR rate at 36%, compared with 60% to 69% in the 2 triple therapy groups. This trial showed the importance of ribavirin in protecting against breakthrough and relapse, even when protease inhibitors are used.

BOCEPREVIR TRIPLE THERAPY
SPRINT–1

This open-label phase 2 trial randomly assigned treatment-naïve patients with geno-type 1 to boceprevir with PegIFN/ribavirin at varying doses and durations with or without a 4-week lead-in with PegIFN and ribavirin dual therapy.[32] All triple therapy groups with boceprevir had higher SVR rates compared with PegIFN/ribavirin alone. In all groups, presence of RVR was a strong positive predictor of SVR, including among patients who were assigned to PegIFN/ribavirin. Nearly two-thirds of patients had undetectable HCV RNA after treatment week 8, following 4 weeks of boceprevir exposure. Of patients who still had detectable HCV RNA by treatment week 12, only 1 ultimately achieved SVR with further therapy.[32]

RESPONSE-GUIDED TRIPLE THERAPY

Response-guided therapy allows for truncation of therapy in patients with an excellent response, and extended therapy in those at higher risk for relapse. Given the increased toxicities and higher dropout rates with triple therapy, response-guided therapy is perhaps even more critical to triple therapy than standard PegIFN/ribavirin therapy. Several phase 3 trials have refined the understanding of response- guided treatment with telaprevir- and boceprevir-based triple therapy.

Telaprevir

Two phase 3 trials, ADVANCE and ILLUMINATE, have augmented knowledge about response-guided therapy with telaprevir therapy. ADVANCE, a phase 3, prospective, randomized, double-blind trial evaluated shortened response-guided therapy with telaprevir in combination with PegIFN/ribavirin in treatment-naïve patients.[33] Patients were randomized to receive either an initial 8 or 12 weeks of telaprevir with PegIFN and ribavirin (T8PR or T12PR) or the standard 48 weeks of PegIFN/ribavirin (PR). Subjects with an extended RVR (eRVR), defined as undetectable HCV RNA at treatment week 4 maintained though treatment week 12, were identified as good responders. In the telaprevir-based groups, those with eRVR were assigned to continue PegIFN/ribavirin to complete 24 weeks of treatment, whereas those without eRVR were assigned to continue PegIFN/ribavirin through treatment week 48. More than half of the patients receiving telaprevir achieved eRVR and were eligible for shortened therapy (57% in the 12-week group, and 58% in the 8-week group). In comparison, only 8% of subjects receiving standard PegIFN/ribavirin achieved eRVR. Both telaprevir-based arms were superior to PegIFN/ribavirin therapy alone in achieving viral eradication (SVR: T12PR, 75%; T8PR, 69%; PR, 44%). Those receiving only 8 weeks of telaprevir had greater virologic failure and developed drug resistance after week 12 compared with the 12-week group.

The ILLUMINATE trial was designed to elucidate whether on-treatment viral kinetics during telaprevir/PegIFN/ribavirin could be used to guide duration of HCV treatment.[34] Treatment-naïve patients with genotype 1 were enrolled, and all were given 12 weeks of telaprevir-based triple therapy, followed by PegIFN and ribavirin treatment of varying duration by group. Among these patients, 65% attained eRVR and were randomized at week 20 to complete either 24 or 48 weeks of total treatment with PegIFN/ribavirin. Those with eRVR had a high SVR rate regardless of the treatment length. The 24-week regimen was not inferior to the 48-week regimen in this favorable subgroup (SVR: 92% for T12PR24 vs 88% for T12PR48). The completion rate was much higher in the 24-week group than the 48-week group (99% vs 74%).

In summary, patients with eRVR have excellent outcome with triple therapy. Response-guided 24-week therapy is not inferior to 48 weeks of therapy in this favorable group with eRVR, and therapy completion rates are improved.

BOCEPREVIR
SPRINT-2

This phase 3, international, randomized, double-blind, placebo-controlled trial investigated the efficacy of boceprevir in combination with PegIFN and ribavirin in treatment-naïve patients with genotype 1, and also investigated the efficacy of response-guided therapy.[35] Patients were randomized to 1 of 3 groups: control (48 weeks of PegIFN/ribavirin), response-guided therapy (4 weeks lead-in with PegIFN/ribavirin followed by boceprevir triple therapy with a response-dependent length of therapy), or fixed-duration therapy (4 weeks lead-in with PegIFN/ribavirin followed by 44 weeks of boceprevir triple therapy). Patients in the response-guided group who achieved and maintained undetectable virus at treatment week 8 through 24 were assigned to 24 total weeks of triple therapy after the 4-week lead-in (for a total treatment duration of 28 weeks), whereas those without an early viral clearance received PegIFN/ribavirin for an additional 20 weeks (for a total treatment duration of 48 weeks). Only 44% had undetectable viral levels between weeks 8 and 24 and were eligible for shortened response-guided therapy. The response-guided and fixed-duration groups had similar SVR rates (63% vs 66%, respectively), and both were superior to standard PegIFN/ribavirin (38%).

Among non-blacks receiving boceprevir, 60% had undetectable virus at week 8, and 47% of all subjects remained negative at week 24. Among these patients with favorable undetectable virus at week 8 and 24, SVR rate was high—97% with 28 weeks therapy and 96% with 48 weeks of therapy. Only 23% of non-blacks and 38% of blacks had a poor response to PegIFN/ribavirin, with a viral decrease of less than $1\text{-}\log_{10}$ IU/mL at 4 weeks after lead-in therapy. Blacks receiving response-guided therapy had slightly lower SVR than the fixed-duration group (42% vs 53%). Overall, however, the addition of boceprevir markedly improved response among this difficult-to-treat group, which has a very poor response to PegIFN/ribavirin dual therapy.

In summary, half of the non-blacks receiving boceprevir cleared HCV RNA by treatment week 8, and 47% had extended undetectable virus and were eligible for a shortened 28-week therapy course. In this favorable group, 24 weeks of triple therapy yielded similar results to 44 weeks of therapy. Insufficient data are available to support response-guided therapy in harder-to-treat patients such as cirrhotics, and therefore FDA recommends against shortened treatment in these patients until more data are gained.[36]

STOPPING RULES

Patients who do not experience rapid viral clearance on triple therapy with DAA are unlikely to attain SVR, even with ongoing treatment. A retrospective data analysis of 3 phase 3 trials with telaprevir triple therapy showed that week 4 viral levels can be used to predict the futility of ongoing treatment, further limiting unnecessary exposure to drug. Findings showed that 1.6% of treatment-naïve patients, 0.7% of prior relapsers, and 14% of prior null responders had HCV RNA levels greater than 1000 IU/mL at week 4.[37] None of these patients attained SVR with ongoing PegIFN/ribavirin treatment, and most (24/25) had reached viral nadir by week 4.[37] Guidelines recommend that telaprevir triple therapy should be discontinued because of futility if the RNA level is greater than 1000 IU/mL at weeks 4 or 12 or detectable at greater than 10 IU/mL at week 24.[36]

Stopping rules for boceprevir take the 4-week PegIFN/ribavirin lead-in into consideration. In patients on boceprevir triple therapy, treatment discontinuation should occur if HCV RNA level is greater than 100 IU/mL at treatment week 12 or detectable at treatment week 24.[36] Stopping therapy protects patients from potential toxicities associated with futile treatment, and also reduces selection of drug-resistant viral variants.

VIRAL ASSAYS

The viral assay used in the telaprevir and boceprevir trials (COBAS Taqman assay; Roche Molecule Systems, version 2.0) has a lower end of quantification of 25 IU/mL, and can detect HCV PCR at 1 to 15 IU/mL. Comparably sensitive assays must be used in clinical practice to have a similar experience, especially considering the fact that the HCV RNA level is the criteria guiding early stopping rules and response-guided therapy. More sensitive assays could misidentify patients and lead to cessation of therapy in patients who would have been eligible for 24-week therapy or continuation of therapy with a different assay.[38]

TREATMENT-EXPERIENCED PATIENTS

Treatment-experienced patients for whom therapy with PegIFN/ribavirin failed have a lower likelihood of having retreatment with PegIFN/ribavirin succeed. Some of these patients, particularly prior null responders, previously had suboptimal response to interferon-based therapy, which also affects response to interferon-based triple therapy with DAA. Three large phase 3 studies have explored this in difficult-to-treat subgroup of patients.

PROVE 3

This phase 2 trial investigated telaprevir with PEG with and without ribavirin at varying lengths of therapy for those previously treated for CHC.[39] These patients for whom prior therapy failed attained higher rates of SVR with triple therapy compared with standard of care, although the arm without ribavirin was inferior. Like PROVE 2, this study again showed the importance of ribavirin in protecting against breakthrough and relapse. Resistance patterns in breakthrough patients were similar to those in treatment-naïve patients. Most patients who discontinued therapy because of the stopping rule had the V36M/R155K double variant, and all but one were genotype 1a.

REALIZE

A study of telaprevir triple therapy in treatment-experienced patients found that the addition of telaprevir significantly improved SVR.[40] Patients were randomized to 1 of 3 groups: 12 weeks of telaprevir triple therapy, with PegIFN/ribavirin through week 48; a lead-in group with 4 weeks of PegIFN/ribavirin followed by 12 weeks of telaprevir triple therapy, then PegIFN/ribavirin through treatment week 48; or control (48 weeks PegIFN/ribavirin). Patients who experienced prior relapse had an excellent response, whereas prior partial responders and prior nonresponders did not have as robust a response and had higher relapse rates. Those receiving telaprevir had a much higher rate of RVR; 70% of group 1 had viral clearance at week 4 compared with 3% of the lead-in group (because they had not yet received telaprevir) and 3% in the control group. By week 8, 93% of group 1 and 89% of the lead-in group had undetectable viral load. Overall SVR for prior relapsers was 83% in group 1 and 88% in the lead-in group compared with 24% in the control group. By week 8, SVR was achieved in 90% to 100% of all prior relapsers with undetectable virus, regardless of which treatment group they were assigned. The group most difficult to treat, the prior nonresponders, still benefitted from triple therapy, with an SVR rate of 29% to 33% compared with 5% with PegIFN/ribavirin.

One Japanese study also confirmed the efficacy of telaprevir triple therapy in difficult-to-treat, treatment-experienced patients with genotype 1b. Patients received 12 weeks of telaprevir in combination with 24 weeks of PegIFN/ribavirin regardless of response. Previous relapsers had a high SVR rate at 88.1%. Prior nonresponders had a lower SVR of 34.4%, but it was improved over that with standard therapy.[41] Prior nonresponders likely need prolonged therapy to improve cure.

RESPOND-2

This trial of boceprevir triple therapy in treatment-experienced patients investigated treatment response in prior partial responders and relapsers, but excluded null responders (those without ≥2-log drop by week 12).[42] The 3 treatment groups included a control arm (48 weeks PegIFN/ribavirin), a fixed-duration arm (4-week lead-in followed by 44 weeks fixed-duration triple therapy), and a response-guided arm (4-week PegIFN/ribavirin lead-in followed by response-guided triple therapy for either 36 or 48 weeks of treatment based on response). In the response-guided arm, those with undetectable HCV RNA at week 8 and 24 continue triple therapy until treatment week 36, whereas those with detectable virus at either time point continued triple therapy until week 48. Of the treatment-experienced patients in the response-guided arm, 46% experienced EVR and were eligible for the 36-week treatment group. Prior relapsers had good outcomes with response-guided and fixed-duration triple therapy, with SVR of 69% and 75%, respectively, compared with 29% with PegIFN/ribavirin. Prior partial responders had 40% and 52% SVR rates with response-guided and fixed-duration therapy, respectively, versus 7% with PegIFN/ribavirin. In summary, treatment-experienced patients have improved rates of viral clearance with triple therapy. Prior relapsers have more success on therapy than prior partial nonresponders, and data on prior null responders are not available for boceprevir.

INTERFERON-FREE THERAPY

All current HCV treatment regimens require interferon, causing many patients with HCV who have contraindications or intolerance to interferon to be ineligible for treatment. Moreover, despite the advances and improved SVR rates with protease inhibitors, treatment-experienced patients who are prior null responders still have low SVR rates, even with the addition of a protease inhibitor. The development of an effective, safe, interferon-free therapy would be of great consequence and result in an increased number of patients eligible for successful treatment.

Many combinations of DAAs are in development. In one phase 1 trial, investigators trialed a combination of tegobuvir and GS-9256, an NS3 protease inhibitor, either as dual therapy, combined with ribavirin, or combined with PegIFN/ribavirin.[43] In the group receiving dual therapy, plasma HCV RNA declined steeply after initiation of treatment, but after 7 days HCV RNA rebounded and resistance-associated variants were detected. Patients who received PegIFN/ribavirin in addition to the 2 DAAs had an RVR rate of 100%.

A new combination therapy with 2 DAAs without PegIFN has achieved SVR in patients with genotype 1b. Noncirrhotic, prior null responders with genotype 1b received once-daily daclatasvir (an NS5A replication complex inhibitor) and asunaprevir (an NS3 protease inhibitor).[44] Ten patients underwent treatment with both drugs, and all who completed the study (9/10) achieved SVR. This dual DAA regimen caused rapid decline in viral load, with mean reductions in baseline viral load of 4.4-$\log_{10}$ IU/mL at week 1, 5.3-$\log_{10}$ IU/mL at week 2, and 5.8-$\log_{10}$ IU/mL from week 4 to end of treatment. At week 4, 40% had undetectable HCV RNA and 90% had levels below the level of quantification. All 9 patients who remained on therapy had undetectable HCV RNA at week 8 and through the end of therapy. Unfortunately, the same regimen was less promising when studied in genotype 1a, a subtype more prone to develop resistance to protease inhibitors and the most common subtype in United States, with only 2 of 9 attaining SVR on dual therapy.[45]

Many other DAAs are under investigation, with the goal of achieving a safe, effective, interferon-free therapy for HCV with minimal toxicities. Discovering a regimen that achieves rapid and sustained viral suppression, and therefore minimizes selection of drug-resistant viral variants, will remain critical in the search for an optimal treatment regimen for chronic hepatitis C infection.

FUTURE IMPLICATIONS

As hepatitis C treatment evolves to potent, all-oral therapy with high SVR rates, the assessment of early viral kinetics will likely be of limited value. Recent phase 2 trials reveal that virtually all subjects will have an RVR, so the predictability becomes less. Even moving to earlier time points (eg, week 2) may offer little discriminative information for determining response-guided therapy if overall SVR rates approach 90%. This problem, however, would be a good one to contemplate. Identifying an optimal duration for large classes of patients (eg, genotype 1a vs 1b) rather than depending on early viral kinetics may prove to be the easiest approach, which would be more easily transferred to less specialized treaters. This article remains to be written.

REFERENCES

1. Choo QL, Kuo G, Weiner AJ, et al. Isolation of a cDNA clone derived from a blood-borne non-A, non-B viral hepatitis genome. Science 1989;244(4902): 359–62.
2. Di Bisceglie AM, Martin P, Kassianides C, et al. Recombinant interferon alfa therapy for chronic hepatitis C. A randomized, double-blind, placebo-controlled trial. N Engl J Med 1989;321(22):1506–10.
3. Davis GL, Balart LA, Schiff ER, et al. Treatment of chronic hepatitis C with recombinant interferon alfa. A multicenter randomized, controlled trial. Hepatitis Interventional Therapy Group. N Engl J Med 1989;321(22):1501–6.
4. Hoofnagle JH, Mullen KD, Jones DB, et al. Treatment of chronic non-A, non-B hepatitis with recombinant human alpha interferon. A preliminary report. N Engl J Med 1986;315(25):1575–8.
5. Blatt LM, Tong MJ, McHutchison JG, et al. Discordance between serum alanine aminotransferase (ALT) and virologic response to IFN-alpha2b in chronic hepatitis C patients with high and low pretreatment serum hepatitis C virus RNA titers. J Interferon Cytokine Res 1998;18(2):75–80.
6. Feld JJ, Hoofnagle JH. Mechanism of action of interferon and ribavirin in treatment of hepatitis C. Nature 2005;436(7053):967–72.
7. Feinberg MB. Changing the natural history of HIV disease. Lancet 1996; 348(9022):239–46.
8. Shindo M, Di Bisceglie AM, Cheung L, et al. Decrease in serum hepatitis C viral RNA during alpha-interferon therapy for chronic hepatitis C. Ann Intern Med 1991;115(9):700–4.
9. Lau JY, Davis GL, Kniffen J, et al. Significance of serum hepatitis C virus RNA levels in chronic hepatitis C. Lancet 1993;341(8859):1501–4.
10. Tsubota A, Chayama K, Ikeda K, et al. Factors predictive of response to interferon-alpha therapy in hepatitis C virus infection. Hepatology 1994;19(5):1088–94.
11. Ge D, Fellay J, Thompson AJ, et al. Genetic variation in IL28B predicts hepatitis C treatment-induced viral clearance. Nature 2009;461(7262):399–401.
12. Layden JE, Layden TJ, Reddy KR, et al. First phase viral kinetic parameters as predictors of treatment response and their influence on the second phase viral decline. J Viral Hepat 2002;9(5):340–5.
13. Bodenheimer HC Jr, Lindsay KL, Davis GL, et al. Tolerance and efficacy of oral ribavirin treatment of chronic hepatitis C: a multicenter trial. Hepatology 1997; 26(2):473–7.
14. Herrmann E, Lee JH, Marinos G, et al. Effect of ribavirin on hepatitis C viral kinetics in patients treated with pegylated interferon. Hepatology 2003;37(6): 1351–8.
15. Management of hepatitis C. NIH Consensus Statement 2012;15(3):1–41.
16. Wiley TE, Briedi L, Lam N, et al. Early HCV RNA values after interferon predict response. Dig Dis Sci 1998;43(10):2169–72.
17. McHutchison JG, Gordon SC, Schiff ER, et al. Interferon alfa-2b alone or in combination with ribavirin as initial treatment for chronic hepatitis C. Hepatitis Interventional Therapy Group. N Engl J Med 1998;339(21):1485–92.
18. Davis GL, Wong JB, McHutchison JG, et al. Early virologic response to treatment with peginterferon alfa-2b plus ribavirin in patients with chronic hepatitis C. Hepatology 2003;38(3):645–52.
19. Fried MW, Shiffman ML, Reddy KR, et al. Peginterferon alfa-2a plus ribavirin for chronic hepatitis C virus infection. N Engl J Med 2002;347(13):975–82.

20. Ghany MG, Strader DB, Thomas DL, et al. Diagnosis, management, and treatment of hepatitis C: an update. Hepatology 2009;49(4):1335–74.

21. Pre-S2 antibodies in hepatitis B. Lancet 1986;2(8521–22):1457–8.

22. Yu JW, Wang GQ, Sun LJ, et al. Predictive value of rapid virological response and early virological response on sustained virological response in HCV patients treated with pegylated interferon alpha-2a and ribavirin. J Gastroenterol Hepatol 2007;22(6):832–6.

23. Hadziyannis SJ, Sette H Jr, Morgan TR, et al. Peginterferon-alpha2a and ribavirin combination therapy in chronic hepatitis C: a randomized study of treatment duration and ribavirin dose. Ann Intern Med 2004;140(5):346–55.

24. Jensen DM, Morgan TR, Marcellin P, et al. Early identification of HCV genotype 1 patients responding to 24 weeks peginterferon alpha-2a (40 kd)/ribavirin therapy. Hepatology 2006;43(5):954–60.

25. Zeuzem S, Buti M, Ferenci P, et al. Efficacy of 24 weeks treatment with peginterferon alfa-2b plus ribavirin in patients with chronic hepatitis C infected with genotype 1 and low pretreatment viremia. J Hepatol 2006;44(1):97–103.

26. Reau N, Satoskar R, Te H, et al. Evaluation of early null response to pegylated interferon and ribavirin as a predictor of therapeutic nonresponse in patients undergoing treatment for chronic hepatitis C. Am J Gastroenterol 2011;106(3):452–8.

27. Reesink HW, Zeuzem S, Weegink CJ, et al. Rapid decline of viral RNA in hepatitis C patients treated with VX-950: a phase Ib, placebo-controlled, randomized study. Gastroenterology 2006;131(4):997–1002.

28. Sarrazin C, Rouzier R, Wagner F, et al. SCH 503034, a novel hepatitis C virus protease inhibitor, plus pegylated interferon alpha-2b for genotype 1 nonresponders. Gastroenterology 2007;132(4):1270–8.

29. Lawitz E, Rodriguez-Torres M, Muir AJ, et al. Antiviral effects and safety of telaprevir, peginterferon alfa-2a, and ribavirin for 28 days in hepatitis C patients. J Hepatol 2008;49(2):163–9.

30. McHutchison JG, Everson GT, Gordon SC, et al. Telaprevir with peginterferon and ribavirin for chronic HCV genotype 1 infection. N Engl J Med 2009;360(18):1827–38.

31. Hezode C, Forestier N, Dusheiko G, et al. Telaprevir and peginterferon with or without ribavirin for chronic HCV infection. N Engl J Med 2009;360(18):1839–50.

32. Kwo PY, Lawitz EJ, McCone J, et al. Efficacy of boceprevir, an NS3 protease inhibitor, in combination with peginterferon alfa-2b and ribavirin in treatment-naive patients with genotype 1 hepatitis C infection (SPRINT-1): an open-label, randomised, multicentre phase 2 trial. Lancet 2010;376(9742):705–16.

33. Jacobson IM, McHutchison JG, Dusheiko G, et al. Telaprevir for previously untreated chronic hepatitis C virus infection. N Engl J Med 2011;364(25):2405–16.

34. Sherman KE, Flamm SL, Afdhal NH, et al. Response-guided telaprevir combination treatment for hepatitis C virus infection. N Engl J Med 2011;365(11):1014–24.

35. Poordad F, McCone J Jr, Bacon BR, et al. Boceprevir for untreated chronic HCV genotype 1 infection. N Engl J Med 2011;364(13):1195–206.

36. Ghany MG, Nelson DR, Strader DB, et al. An update on treatment of genotype 1 chronic hepatitis C virus infection: 2011 practice guideline by the American Association for the Study of Liver Diseases. Hepatology 2011;54(4):1433–44.

37. Jacobson IM, Bartels D, Gritz L, et al. Futility Rules in Telaprevir Combination Treatment. J Hepatol 2012;56(Suppl 2):S24.

38. Fevery B, Susser S, Cloherty G, et al. Comparison of two quantitative HCV RNA assays in samples from patients treated with a protease inhibitor - based therapy: implications for response guided therapy. J Hepatol 2012;56(Suppl 2):S26.

39. McHutchison JG, Manns MP, Muir AJ, et al. Telaprevir for previously treated chronic HCV infection. N Engl J Med 2010;362(14):1292–303.
40. Zeuzem S, Andreone P, Pol S, et al. Telaprevir for retreatment of HCV infection. N Engl J Med 2011;364(25):2417–28.
41. Hayashi N, Okanoue T, Tsubouchi H, et al. Efficacy and safety of telaprevir, a new protease inhibitor, for difficult-to-treat patients with genotype 1 chronic hepatitis C. J Viral Hepat 2012;19(2):e134–42.
42. Bacon BR, Gordon SC, Lawitz E, et al. Boceprevir for previously treated chronic HCV genotype 1 infection. N Engl J Med 2011;364(13):1207–17.
43. Zeuzem S, Buggisch P, Agarwal K, et al. The protease inhibitor, GS-9256, and non-nucleoside polymerase inhibitor tegobuvir alone, with ribavirin, or pegylated interferon plus ribavirin in hepatitis C. Hepatology 2012;55(3):749–58.
44. Chayama K, Takahashi S, Toyota J, et al. Dual therapy with the nonstructural protein 5A inhibitor, daclatasvir, and the nonstructural protein 3 protease inhibitor, asunaprevir, in hepatitis C virus genotype 1b-infected null responders. Hepatology 2012;55(3):742–8.
45. Lok A, Gardiner D, Lawitz E, et al. Quadruple therapy with BMS-790052, BMS-650032, and peg-IFN/RBV for 24 weeks results in 100% SVR12 in HCV genotype 1 null responders (abstract). J Hepatol 2011;54(Suppl 1):1356.

Approach to the Treatment-naïve Patient with HCV Genotype 1 Infection

Andrew J. Muir, MD, MHS

KEYWORDS

- HCV genotype 1 • Boceprevir • Telaprevir • Treatment-naïve patients

KEY POINTS

- Protease inhibitor regimens lead to substantial increases in treatment response for treatment naïve genotype 1 patients compared to peginterferon-α and ribavirin.
- Protease inhibitors must be given in combination with peginterferon-α and ribavirin.
- Response guided therapy algorithms for the protease inhibitor regimens allow patients with early response to shorten the duration of therapy to 24 to 28 weeks.
- New adverse events with protease inhibitors include anemia with both boceprevir and telaprevir and severe rash with telaprevir.

In May 2011, the protease inhibitors boceprevir and telaprevir were approved in combination with peginterferon-α and ribavirin for the treatment of genotype 1 chronic hepatitis C virus (HCV) infection in the United States. These regimens brought substantial improvements in sustained virologic response rates (SVR), especially for treatment-naïve patients. This article reviews the approach to therapy with these genotype 1 treatment naïve patients.

ELIGIBILITY FOR PROTEASE INHIBITOR COMBINATION THERAPY

For patients with genotype 1 infection, the new standard of care is peginterferon-α, ribavirin, and a protease inhibitor. Although there has been tremendous excitement with the improved responses of the protease inhibitors, eligibility for therapy remains driven largely by the adverse event profile of peginterferon-α and ribavirin. Peginterferon-α causes severe flulike symptoms and is contraindicated in patients with severe comorbidities, such as chronic obstructive pulmonary disease or coronary artery disease or a history of decompensated cirrhosis, including history of variceal hemorrhage, ascites, and hepatic encephalopathy.[1] Peginterferon-α is associated with

Division of Gastroenterology, Duke Clinical Research Institute, Duke University School of Medicine, Room 0311 Terrace Level 2400 Pratt Street, Durham, NC 27715, USA
E-mail address: andrew.muir@duke.edu

Infect Dis Clin N Am 26 (2012) 893–901
http://dx.doi.org/10.1016/j.idc.2012.08.012
0891-5520/12/$ – see front matter © 2012 Published by Elsevier Inc.

id.theclinics.com

depressive symptoms, including suicidal ideation and is not recommended in patients with major uncontrolled depressive illness or other forms of severe mental illness. Peginterferon-α may exacerbate autoimmune disorders and is also contraindicated in recipients of heart, lung, and kidney transplants. Peginterferon-α causes bone marrow suppression. Patients with low blood counts would likely need dose reductions or early discontinuations. Ribavirin causes hemolytic anemia and is renally cleared. Patients with baseline anemia and renal impairment have increased risk of adverse events with ribavirin.

When considering new contraindications with the protease inhibitors, additional anemia attributable to both protease inhibitors was observed in the clinical trials. Patients being considered for treatment need evaluation of baseline anemia or marginal hemoglobin levels before initiation of therapy.[2,3]

MAJOR PUBLISHED STUDIES OF BOCEPREVIR AND TELAPREVIR
Boceprevir

Lessons from phase 1 and 2 studies
Early in the development of boceprevir, resistance was observed quickly with monotherapy.[4] As a result, approaches were studied to reduce resistance, including the lead-in strategy in which patients receive peginterferon-α and ribavirin for 4 weeks before the addition of boceprevir. In the phase 2 Serine Protease Inhibitor Therapy (SPRINT)-1 trial, which included arms with and without lead-in, viral breakthrough occurred in 19 (9%) of 210 patients without the lead-in compared with 9 (4%, $P = .057$) of 206 patients with lead-in.[5] The lead-in strategy was ultimately used in phase 3. The other major lesson from phase 2 was the importance of ribavirin. To try to reduce the anemia and side effects with treatment, one arm of the study included a low dose of ribavirin at 400 to 1000 mg in a weigh-based approach compared with 800 to 1400 mg in the other arms. This lower ribavirin dose arm achieved SVR in only 36% of patients with viral breakthrough in 27%. As a result, the phase 3 study arms included full-dose ribavirin.

Boceprevir

Phase 3 clinical trial
The phase 3 treatment-naïve study for boceprevir was called SPRINT-2.[3] This was a randomized, double-blind, placebo-controlled trial with 3 arms, including a control arm of peginterferon-α and ribavirin. Because of the lower response rate previously observed in African American patients, this study also had separate cohorts of black and nonblack patients.[6] All patients in the boceprevir-containing arms received a 4-week "lead-in" phase of pegylated interferon plus ribavirin dual therapy before the addition of boceprevir. In the "response-guided therapy" (RGT) arm patients who achieved an undetectable HCV RNA from weeks 8 to 24 (ie, "early responders") stopped all treatment at week 28. Those who did not achieve a nondetectable viral load at week 8, but did achieve viral suppression at 24 weeks (ie, "late responders") completed an additional 20 weeks of pegylated interferon plus ribavirin therapy for a total of 48 weeks of treatment. In the third group, patients completed 44 weeks of triple therapy after the 4-week lead-in phase, even if they were an early responder. Treatment was discontinued for any patient who did not achieve viral suppression by 24 weeks.

The SVR rates, which are detailed in **Table 1**, were significantly improved with the addition of boceprevir, compared with dual therapy alone, in both black and nonblack patients. The results also demonstrated excellent virologic outcomes for early responders (nondetectable HCV RNA at week 8) regardless of treatment duration, supporting the utility of an RGT approach (SVR rates 88% vs 90%, respectively). As

Table 1
Response rates from the boceprevir phase 3 naïve trial

	Non-Black RGT	Non-Black 48 Weeks	Black RGT	Black 48 Weeks
SVR	211/316 (67%)	213/311 (68%)	26/52 (50%)	36/55 (65%)
Relapse	21/232 (9%)	18/230 (8%)	3/25 (12%)	6/35 (17%)
% eligible for shortened duration (undetectable week 8–24)	147/316 (46%)	N/A	15/52 (29%)	N/A
SVR if undetectable week 8–24	143/147 (97%)	N/A	13/15 (87%)	N/A
Bridging fibrosis/cirrhosis	13/26 (50%)	18/36 (50%)	1/8 (12%)	4/6 (67%)

Abbreviations: RGT, response-guided therapy; SVR, sustained virologic response.
  Data from Poordad F, McCone J Jr, Bacon BR, et al. Boceprevir for untreated chronic HCV genotype 1 infection. N Engl J Med 2011;364(13):1195–206.

demonstrated in **Table 1**, 143 (97%) of 147 early responders in the nonblack cohort and 13 (87%) of 15 in the black cohort achieved SVR with 28 weeks of treatment. A major question to guide clinical decision making is the likelihood of SVR in patients with cirrhosis. In the SPRINT-2 study, the SVR rate for both cohorts among patients with cirrhosis was 41% (14/34) in the boceprevir response-guided therapy arm and 52% (22/42) in the boceprevir 48-week arm, suggesting potential benefit of longer treatment duration among those with advanced liver disease. Among patients without cirrhosis, no difference was observed in the response-guided therapy arm (213/319, 67%) or the boceprevir-containing 48-week treatment arm (211/313, 67%); lack of cirrhosis was a predictor of SVR.

Telaprevir

Lessons from phase 1 and 2 studies
The early development program with telaprevir revealed the development of viral resistance with monotherapy, as was seen with boceprevir, and therefore telaprevir was developed in combination with peginterferon-α and ribavirin.[7] From an early point, the telaprevir program focused on triple therapy with peginterferon-α, ribavirin, and telaprevir for 12 weeks with further evaluation of the role of ribavirin and the need for additional peginterferon-α and ribavirin. The Protease Inhibition for Viral Evaluation (PROVE)-1 trial was a phase 2 trial in which all patients received 12 weeks of the triple combination.[8] One group received no further treatment whereas the other 2 intervention groups received 12 and 36 more weeks of peginterferon-α and ribavirin. In the 12-week therapy arm, only 6 (35%) of 17 patients achieved SVR; this failed strategy that did not move to phase 3 development. The PROVE-2 study was a phase 2 trial conducted in Europe that also examined the duration of treatment but included one intervention arm without ribavirin.[9] This ribavirin-free approach led to SVR in 28 (36%) of 78 patients with relapse in 22 (48%) of 46 patients, illustrating the importance of ribavirin, which was included in the 2 phase 3 trials.

Phase 3
For treatment-naïve patients, the 2 phase 3 trials were A New Direction in HCV Care: A Study of Treatment Naïve Hepatitis C patients with Telaprevir (ADVANCE) and Illustrating the Effects of Combination Therapy with Telaprevir (ILLUMINATE).[2,10] During the phase 2 studies, a perception developed that the rash associated with telaprevir

occurred around or after week 8. If so, shortening the duration of telaprevir exposure might maximize efficacy and minimize the adverse event. Thus, the ADVANCE trial was designed to compare 8 and 12 weeks of the triple combination of peginterferon-α, ribavirin, and telaprevir followed by a tail of peginterferon-α and ribavirin. In the end, the rates of rash were comparable in both arms, whereas the SVR rates were numerically higher in the 12-week arm (**Table 2**). However, the reasonable SVR rates with the 8-week triple combination suggest that early discontinuation of telaprevir for an adverse event with continuation of peginterferon-α and ribavirin can be an effective strategy.

The ILLUMINATE trial focused on the ability to shorten therapy with the telaprevir combination therapy.[10] If patients achieved an extended rapid virologic response (eRVR), defined as undetectable HCV RNA at weeks 4 and 12, patients were randomized to stop treatment at week 24 or continue pegylated interferon plus ribavirin to week 48. Of the 540 patients in the study, 352 (65%) achieved eRVR, and 322 patients were randomized to 24 or 48 weeks of total treatment duration. The SVR rates were similar whether these patients were treated for 24 weeks (149/162, 92%) or 48 weeks (140/160, 88%), thus providing the rationale to shorten the treatment duration among early virologic responders who do not have underlying cirrhosis.

TREATMENT ALGORITHMS: RESPONSE-GUIDED THERAPY FOR GENOTYPE 1 PATIENTS
Algorithms

The treatment algorithms for the protease inhibitor regimens have a number of goals. For patients who respond early to the medications, the phase 3 studies demonstrated that SVR can be achieved with 24 weeks of treatment with telaprevir and 28 weeks with boceprevir. For patients with cirrhosis, response-guided therapy is not an option, and instead 48 weeks of treatment is required to maximize chances of cure. Given the development of resistance among many patients who fail the protease inhibitor combinations, the algorithms also stop treatment early for these patients to minimize the duration of treatment after the emergence of the resistant variants. These algorithms and futility rules are similar to the designs of the phase 3 trials and are outlined in **Fig. 1**. The algorithms include decisions based on attainment of an undetectable

Table 2 Response rates from the telaprevir phase 3 naïve trials			
	Advance T12PR	**ADVANCE T8PR**	**ILLUMINATE T12PR**
SVR	271/363 (75%)	250/364 (69%)	389/540 (72%)
Relapse	27/314 (9%)	28/295 (9%)	37/469 (8%)
% eligible for shortened duration (eRVR)	212/363 (58%)	207/364 (57%)	352/540 (65%)
SVR if eRVR and 24 weeks duration	189/212 (89%)	171/207 (83%)	149/162 (92%)
Bridging fibrosis or cirrhosis	45/73 (62%)	24/73 (33%)	94/149 (63%)
African American/Black	16/26 (62%)	7/28 (25%)	44/73 (60%)

Abbreviations: eRVR, undetectable HCV RNA at weeks 4 and 12; SVR, sustained virologic response; T8PR, 8 weeks of telaprevir, peginterferon-α, ribavirin and then 16–40 weeks peginterferon-α, ribavirin; T12PR, 12 weeks of telaprevir, peginterferon-α, ribavirin and then 12–36 weeks peginterferon-α, ribavirin.

Data from Jacobson IM, McHutchison JG, Dusheiko G, et al. Telaprevir for previously untreated chronic hepatitis C virus infection. N Engl J Med 2011;364(25):2405–16; and Sherman KE, Flamm SL, Afdhal NH, et al. Response-guided telaprevir combination treatment for hepatitis C virus infection. N Engl J Med 2011;365(11):1014–24.

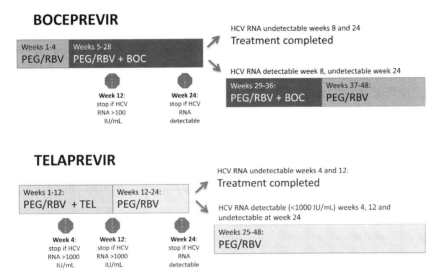

Fig. 1. HCV protease inhibitor algorithms for treatment naïve genotype 1 infection.

HCV RNA level, and the Food and Drug Administration (FDA) recommends use of an assay with a lower limit of HCV RNA quantification less than or equal to 25 IU/mL and a limit of HCV RNA detection of approximately 10 to 15 IU/mL.

The boceprevir algorithm begins with the lead-in of peginterferon-α and ribavirin for 4 weeks with the addition of boceprevir to the combination in week 5.[11] The duration of treatment depends on when viremia is suppressed. If patients have undetectable HCV RNA at weeks 8 and 24, patients should stop treatment at week 28. If HCV RNA is detectable at week 8, but is undetectable by week 24, the patient requires treatment for 48 weeks (triple combination until week 36 with 12 additional weeks of peginterferon-α and ribavirin without boceprevir). Treatment is discontinued if HCV RNA is greater than 100 IU/mL at week 12 or detectable at week 24.

In the telaprevir algorithm, patients start peginterferon-α, ribavirin, and telaprevir at week 1 and continue for 12 weeks.[12] If patients have HCV RNA greater than 1000 IU/mL at week 4 or week 12, they stop all treatment. If patients achieve eRVR (undetectable HCV RNA at weeks 4 and 12), they receive 12 more weeks of peginterferon-α and ribavirin and then stop all therapy at week 24. For patients who do not achieve eRVR but pass the futility rules, they will receive 36 more weeks of peginterferon-α and ribavirin. These patients would also stop therapy if HCV RNA is detectable at week 24.

Resistance

The introduction of the protease inhibitors has brought the issue of viral resistance into the clinical practice of HCV for the first time. Both protease inhibitors lead to resistance with monotherapy, and regimens lacking ribavirin or using low-dose ribavirin led to increased resistance in the phase 2 studies.[4,5,7,9] As a result, treatment regimens require full-dose ribavirin initially, and patients need to be educated about the importance of adherence to all medications to decrease the likelihood of resistance. Adherence to the protease inhibitors can be especially challenging given the dosing requirements. Both protease inhibitors must be taken every 7 to 9 hours, and patients should develop a reminder strategy to avoid missing or delaying doses.[11,12] Because of food effects that increase exposure, boceprevir must be taken with a meal or light snack, and telaprevir should be taken with 20 g of fat. Drug-drug interactions with the protease inhibitors can also affect exposure. Both protease inhibitors are substrates and inhibitors of cytochrome P450 3A, and some drugs therefore will lead to reduced levels of the protease inhibitor.[11,12] Medication reconciliation and a strategy to evaluate for drug-drug interactions are also key aspects of care for patients receiving HCV treatment.

The use of the lead-in strategy with boceprevir has provided insight into the role of the peginterferon-α and ribavirin backbone in preventing the development of resistance. In the phase 3 SPRINT-2 trial with boceprevir, the magnitude of the reduction in HCV RNA at week 4 predicted the development of resistant variants.[3] In the response-guided therapy group, only 10 (4%) of 232 patients with a reduction of more than 1 log in HCV RNA at 4 weeks developed resistance. In contrast, 49 (52%) of 95 patients with a reduction of less than 1 log in HCV RNA developed resistance. These data highlight the importance of the interferon responsiveness of the patient in the development of resistance and the success of protease inhibitor combination therapy.

INTERLEUKIN-28B

While the phase 3 protease inhibitor trials were ongoing, a genome-wide association study reported that a single nucleotide polymorphism near the interleukin-28B (IL28B) gene was associated with treatment response.[13] This discovery was made during a trial of treatment with peginterferon-α and ribavirin, and one natural question was the impact of the IL28B genotype on outcomes with protease inhibitor combinations. Analyses from the SPRINT-2 (boceprevir) and ADVANCE (telaprevir) trials were retrospectively performed, and the results are summarized in **Fig. 2**.[14,15] The ADVANCE analysis included only the white patients from the study. The findings demonstrate that all patients benefit from protease inhibitors regardless of their IL28B genotypes, although the patients with favorable IL28B genotype have higher SVR rates. Patients with the favorable IL28B genotype are also more likely to qualify for shortened duration

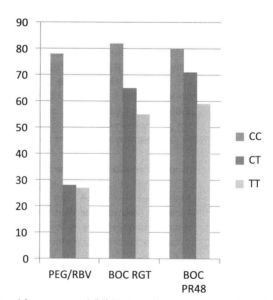

Fig. 2. SVR rates with protease inhibitor combinations according to IL28B genotype rs12979860. PEG, peginterferon alfa; RBV, ribavirin; RGT, response guided therapy; BOC, boceprevir; PR48, peginterferon alfa and ribavirin for 48 weeks.

of treatment. As discussed in the recent update of the American Association for the Study of Liver Diseases guideline, IL28B is not required for HCV treatment but can be useful to patients if the likelihood of SVR or shortened duration of therapy would affect patient decisions regarding treatment.[1]

SAFETY

Given the need for protease inhibitors to be given in combination with peginterferon-α and ribavirin, the adverse event profile remains dominated by the effects of peginterferon-α. The phase 3 studies with the protease inhibitors did reveal some adverse events that were attributable to the protease inhibitors.

Anemia

Anemia is a well-known complication of HCV therapy with bone marrow suppression from peginterferon-α and hemolysis from ribavirin, but treatment with the protease inhibitor combinations leads to further reduction in hemoglobin by an unclear mechanism. Comparisons between boceprevir and telaprevir are challenging from the phase 3 trials for a number of reasons. The boceprevir SPRINT-2 study allowed the use of erythropoietin for the management of anemia, but the telaprevir ADVANCE and ILLUMINATE studies required dose reduction of ribavirin and did not allow erythropoietin-stimulating agents.[2,3,10] The studies reported anemia in different ways, but both reported clear increases in anemia events compared with the control groups of peginterferon-α and ribavirin without a protease inhibitor. In the SPRINT-2 study, anemia was reported as an adverse event in 49% of patients receiving the boceprevir regiment compared with 29% in the controls. Erythropoietin was used in 43% of patients in the boceprevir groups, and 20 (2.7%) of 734 patients in the boceprevir groups required transfusions of packed red blood cells. In the telaprevir ADVANCE study, dose reductions and potential discontinuation of treatment were required, and 1% of patients in the T12PR group (12 weeks of telaprevir, peginterferon-α, and ribavirin, and then 12–36 weeks peginterferon-α and ribavirin) and 3% of patients in the T8PR group (8 weeks of telaprevir, peginterferon-α, and ribavirin, and then 16–40 weeks peginterferon-α and ribavirin) discontinued all treatment because of anemia. Serious adverse events attributable to anemia occurred in 18 (2.5%) of 727 patients receiving telaprevir, and 34 (4.7%) of 727 patients in the telaprevir groups received transfusions of packed red blood cells.

Anemia is therefore a common adverse event in treatment with protease inhibitor regimens. Triggers for the management of anemia include hemoglobin less than 10 g per deciliter or a reduction of 3 g per deciliter in patients with underlying heart disease. Close monitoring in the first few weeks of protease inhibitor therapy is critical to avoid severe anemia. Ribavirin dose reduction is the strategy recommended by the FDA for the management of anemia, and erythropoietin-stimulating agents are not approved for this indication.[11,12] Similar virologic outcomes have been achieved with and without the use of erythropoietin-stimulating agents with the protease inhibitor regimens. If providers and patients elect to use these agents in the management of anemia, the boceprevir program data demonstrate the experience with anemia with their use. The telaprevir program data would suggest that ribavirin dose reduction is a very reasonable strategy that still leads to high SVR rates.

Gastrointestinal Adverse Events

In the boceprevir program, dysgeusia or abnormal taste was more common in patients receiving boceprevir compared with patients in the control group.[11] In the telaprevir program, a variety of anorectal adverse events that included hemorrhoidal symptoms and anorectal burning were more common in patients receiving telaprevir.[12] These adverse events did not lead to discontinuation of treatment but may require symptomatic management.

Rash

In the phase 2 studies with telaprevir, a maculopapular rash emerged and was associated with treatment, and the PROVE-1 phase 2 study was amended to provide grading criteria.[8] Interestingly, 41% of patients in the control group not receiving telaprevir in PROVE-1 reported rash, and 40% were mild or moderate. In the telaprevir arms, 53% to 61% of patients developed rash, and 5% to 9% were severe. Although uncommon, Stevens-Johnson Syndrome and Drug Reaction Eosinophilia and Systemic Symptoms (DRESS) have been reported with telaprevir.[12] Seven percent of patients in the telaprevir arms in PROVE-1 discontinued treatment because of rash.

As a result, a rash management plan was developed for phase 3 and mimics the current management recommendations.[2,12] Patients with mild to moderate rash are monitored closely and given symptomatic treatments. If the rash progresses to become generalized or develops vesicles, bullae, or ulcerations, telaprevir must be discontinued. Assuming the rash is not Stevens-Johnson Syndrome or DRESS, treatment with peginterferon-α and ribavirin can be continued as long as the rash improves after discontinuing the telaprevir. If there is worsening or no improvement of the rash, all medications should be discontinued. In PROVE-1, 7% of patients discontinued all treatment because of rash.[8] With the rash management plan in place in the phase 3 ADVANCE trial, 7% of patients discontinued telaprevir because of rash but only 1.4% discontinued all treatment.[2] The current rash management guidelines allow patients to gain the benefit from as many weeks of telaprevir as possible but avoid discontinuing all medications to help them achieve SVR.

SUMMARY

The addition of the protease inhibitors boceprevir and telaprevir to peginterferon-α and ribavirin has been a tremendous step forward for genotype 1–naïve patients. For some patients, the protease inhibitors offer the opportunity to shorten therapy from the typical 48 weeks down to 24 or 28 weeks. Challenges remain given that boceprevir and telaprevir must be given in combination with peginterferon-α and ribavirin, and many patients are not eligible because of the adverse event profiles of these medications. Boceprevir and telaprevir bring new adverse events forward, with the rash with telaprevir and the anemia with both medications requiring close monitoring and new management strategies.

REFERENCES

1. Ghany MG, Nelson DR, Strader DB, et al. An update on treatment of genotype 1 chronic hepatitis C virus infection: 2011 practice guideline by the American Association for the Study of Liver Diseases. Hepatology 2011;54(4):1433–44.
2. Jacobson IM, McHutchison JG, Dusheiko G, et al. Telaprevir for previously untreated chronic hepatitis C virus infection. N Engl J Med 2011;364(25): 2405–16.
3. Poordad F, McCone J Jr, Bacon BR, et al. Boceprevir for untreated chronic HCV genotype 1 infection. N Engl J Med 2011;364(13):1195–206.

4. Susser S, Welsch C, Wang Y, et al. Characterization of resistance to the protease inhibitor boceprevir in hepatitis C virus-infected patients. Hepatology 2009;50(6): 1709–18.

5. Kwo PY, Lawitz EJ, McCone J, et al. Efficacy of boceprevir, an NS3 protease inhibitor, in combination with peginterferon alfa-2b and ribavirin in treatment-naive patients with genotype 1 hepatitis C infection (SPRINT-1): an open-label, randomised, multicentre phase 2 trial. Lancet 2010;376(9742):705–16.

6. Muir AJ, Bornstein JD, Killenberg PG. Peginterferon alfa-2b and ribavirin for the treatment of chronic hepatitis C in African blacks and non-Hispanic whites. N Engl J Med 2004;350:2265–71.

7. Kieffer TL, Sarrazin C, Miller JS, et al. Telaprevir and pegylated interferon-alpha-2a inhibit wild-type and resistant genotype 1 hepatitis C virus replication in patients. Hepatology 2007;46(3):631–9.

8. McHutchison JG, Everson GT, Gordon SC, et al. Telaprevir with peginterferon and ribavirin for chronic HCV genotype 1 infection. N Engl J Med 2009;360:1827–38.

9. Hézode C, Forestier N, Dusheiko G, et al. Telaprevir and peginterferon with or without ribavirin for chronic HCV infection. N Engl J Med 2009;360(18):1839–50.

10. Sherman KE, Flamm SL, Afdhal NH, et al. Response-guided telaprevir combination treatment for hepatitis C virus infection. N Engl J Med 2011;365(11):1014–24.

11. Victrelis (boceprevir) prescribing information. 2012. Available at: http://www.accessdata.fda.gov/scripts/cder/drugsatfda/. Accessed May 20, 2012.

12. Incivek (telaprevir) prescribing information. 2012. Available at: http://www.accessdata.fda.gov/scripts/cder/drugsatfda/. Accessed May 20, 2012.

13. Ge D, Fellay J, Thompson AJ, et al. Genetic variation in IL28B predicts hepatitis C treatment-induced viral clearance. Nature 2009;461:399–401.

14. Poordad F, Bronowicki JP, Gordon SC, et al. IL28B polymorphism predicts virologic response in patients with hepatitis C genotype 1 treated with boceprevir (BOC) combination therapy. J Hepatol 2011;54(Suppl 1):S6.

15. Jacobson IM, Catlett I, Marcellin P, et al. Telaprevir substantially improved SVR rates across all IL28B genotypes in the advance trial. J Hepatol 2011;54(Suppl 1):S542–3.

Approach to the Treatment-Experienced Patient with Hepatitis C Virus Genotype 1 Infection

Jennifer A. Flemming, MD, Norah A. Terrault, MD, MPH*

KEYWORDS

- Protease inhibitor • Hepatitis C • Antiviral • Treatment-experienced • Relapser
- Partial responder • Null responder • Systemic vascular resistance

KEY POINTS

- Recently US Food and Drug Administration-approved protease inhibitors (PIs) boceprevir and telaprevir, added to peginterferon and ribavirin (Peg-IFN/RBV), significantly increase sustained virologic response rates in patients with hepatitis C virus genotype 1 infection and history of previous non-sustained response to Peg-IFN/RBV.
- Expected sustained virologic response rates with PI triple therapy are highly dependent on the patient's previous on-treatment response and underlying degree of liver fibrosis.
- Prior relapsers are excellent candidates for retreatment with PI triple therapy and often qualify for response-guided therapy, with a shorter duration of treatment used in those with early viral suppression. In contrast, response-guided therapy has limited use in treatment-experienced patients with prior partial and null responses.
- Virologic response to a 4-week Peg-IFN/RBV lead-in period can help guide treatment decisions in patients with an unknown previous response to Peg-IFN/RBV.
- Since a substantial proportion of previously treated patients will not achieve SVR when retreated with PI triple therapy, the need for new therapies in these patients remains high.

INTRODUCTION

Approximately 60% of patients with hepatitis C virus (HCV) genotype 1 (GT1) infection who previously received a course of antiviral therapy with peginterferon (Peg-IFN) and ribavirin (RBV) will not achieve sustained clearance of virus.[1] These nonsustained responders are distinguished from peg-IFN/RBV intolerant patients who were unable to complete a course of therapy at target doses of the drugs, classically defined as

Department of Medicine, Viral Hepatitis Center, University of California San Francisco, Room S-357, 513 Parnassus Avenue, San Francisco, CA 94143, USA
* Corresponding author.
E-mail address: norah.terrault@ucsf.edu

Infect Dis Clin N Am 26 (2012) 903–915
http://dx.doi.org/10.1016/j.idc.2012.08.008
0891-5520/12/$ – see front matter © 2012 Elsevier Inc. All rights reserved.

taking at least 80% of the treatment dose for at least 80% of the proposed treatment duration. Nonsustained responders comprise a heterogeneous group. Four subtypes of prior treatment response are recognized (**Fig. 1**). Patients are considered to have relapse if their HCV RNA is undetectable at the end of treatment but positive after treatment is stopped. Partial response is defined as having at least a 2-log drop in HCV RNA at week 12 of therapy but failure to become undetectable by week 24 of treatment. Null response is defined by a failure to achieve a 2-log drop in HCV RNA at week 12 of Peg-IFN/RBV. Finally, virologic breakthrough is when a patient has an undetectable HCV RNA during treatment but then becomes persistently HCV RNA positive while still on therapy. The sustained virologic response (SVR) rates for treatment-experienced patients re-treated with a second course of Peg-IFN/RBV ranges from only 6% to 23% depending on their prior treatment response, with the highest rates of response seen in prior relapsers.[2–5] Given these poor results, the need for new therapies for these treatment-experienced patients is high.

The approval of the first NS3/4A protease inhibitors (PIs), boceprevir (BOC) and telaprevir (TPV), in combination with Peg-IFN/RBV for treatment of GT1 infection in prior nonsustained responders of Peg-IFN/RBV therapy gave new hope for treatment-experienced patients. Moreover, the concept of response guided-therapy (RGT)—with duration of treatment influenced by the achievement of specific virologic benchmarks—gained prominence as a treatment strategy. With PI triple therapy, patients who achieved HCV RNA undetectability early in treatment (weeks 4–8, depending on the PI used) were potentially eligible for shorter duration treatment (24–28 weeks), whereas patients who did not achieve this early virologic response were treated for 48 weeks.

However, as highlighted in this article, a significant proportion of treatment-experienced patients will not achieve SVR with PI triple therapy, and so the need for alternative therapies for these patients remains high. The aim of this article is to provide a critical evaluation of the available data, highlighting the knowledge gaps and providing a practical framework for making treatment decisions in treatment-experienced GT1 patients with currently approved drugs.

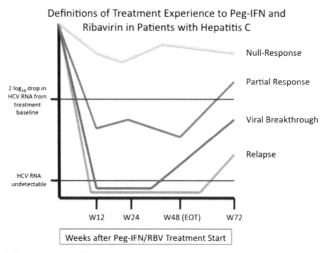

Fig. 1. Four different types of virologic nonresponse to previous treatment with Peg-IFN and RBV in patients with chronic hepatitis C.

OVERVIEW OF CLINICAL TRIALS OF TPV AND BOC IN TREATMENT-EXPERIENCED PATIENTS

The key aspects of the clinical trials evaluating BOC and TPV in treatment-experienced patients are listed in **Table 1**.

Boceprevir

Randomized controlled trials (BOC)

RESPOND-2 was the pivotal phase 3 trial comparing triple therapy with BOC 800 mg 3 times daily (every 7–9 hours), Peg-IFN alfa-2b at 1.5 μg/kg/wk and weight-based RBV (600–1400 mg/d) to Peg-IFN/RBV alone in 403 treatment-experienced patients with chronic HCV GT1 from 80 sites in North America and Europe (**Fig. 2**).[6] Of note, previous null responders were not included in this study. Patients were stratified by

Table 1
Summary of pivotal trials of TPV triple therapy and BOC triple therapy in treatment-experienced GT1 patients

Study	TPV		BOC		
	REALIZE[9]	Muir et al[11]	RESPOND-2[6]	PROVIDE,[8a]	Flamm et al[12a]
Type of Peg-IFN	alfa-2a	alfa-2a	alfa-2b	alfa-2b	alfa-2a
RBV dose (mg/d)	1000 or 1200	1000 or 1200	600–1400	600–1400	1000 or 1200
Lead-in	Yes (1 arm)	No	Yes	Yes	No
RGT	Yes	No	Yes	No	No
Total # of patients	663	117	403	168	201
Mean age, y	51	50	53	52	–
Male sex, %	70	69	87	67	70
African American, %	5	8	13	–	–
HCV Subgenotype, %					
1a	45	59	58	61	–
1b	45	32	42	39	–
Fibrosis stage, %					
0–2	54	62	74	–	–
3–4	47	38	19	–	–
Cirrhosis	25	9	12	10	16
SVR rates by prior response					
Relapse, %	83–88	97	69–75	68[b]	70
Partial response, %	54–59	55	40–52	68[b]	–
Null response, %	29–33	56	–	40	47
Predictors of SVR					
Peg-IFN/RBV lead-in	✔		✔		✔
eRVR			✔		
Baseline fibrosis	✔		✔		
Baseline viral load	✔		✔		
Sub-genotype (1b/1a)	✔		✔		
Body mass index (≤25 vs >30)			✔		
Age <40	✔				
Nonblack race	✔				
Statin use	✔				

[a] Studies presented in abstract form, and complete data not available.
[b] Relapsers and partial responders summarized together.

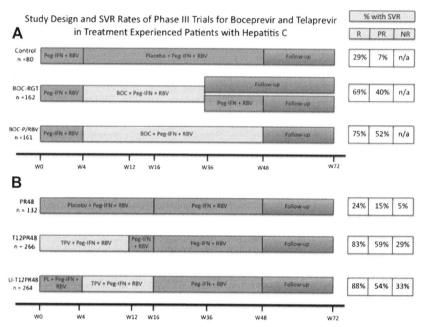

Fig. 2. Summary of the phase 3 trials for protease inhibitors with rates of SVR based on prior treatment response. (*A*) Results from RESPOND-2 with BOC. (*B*) Results from REALIZE for TPV. *Abbreviations:* NR, nonresponse; PR, partial response; R, relapse.

previous treatment response (relapse vs partial response) and subgenotype (1a or 1b). The treatment duration was 48 weeks, but an RGT approach was evaluated. All patients received a lead-in of Peg-IFN/RBV alone for the first 4 weeks. In the control Group 1, 80 subjects received placebo/Peg-IFN/RBV for an additional 44 weeks. In Group 2 RGT, 162 received BOC/Peg-IFN/RBV for 36 weeks, with those who were HCV RNA undetectable at weeks 8 and 12 stopping treatment at week 36, whereas those who were HCV RNA detectable at week 8, but negative at week 12, receiving an additional 12 weeks of Peg-IFN/RBV after triple therapy was completed, for a total of 48 weeks of therapy. In Group 3, 161 subjects received BOC/Peg-IFN/RBV for 44 weeks after the 4-week lead in phase of PEG/RBV. SVR was assessed 24 weeks after treatment stopped. Baseline characteristics of the treated patients are noteworthy for the low proportion of patients with cirrhosis and higher than usual percentage of African Americans (see **Table 1**).

Compared with the Peg-IFN/RBV arm, the rates of SVR were significantly better in the BOC-containing arms, with overall SVR rates of 22% versus 59% (RGT BOC therapy) versus 66% (44 weeks BOC therapy) (*P*<.001) (see **Fig. 2**). Independent predictors of SVR in BOC-treated patients included lower baseline fibrosis, previous relapse (vs partial response), subgenotype 1b, lower body mass index and lower (<800,000 IU/mL) baseline viral load.[7] However, the strongest independent predictor of SVR was lead-in response to Peg-IFN/RBV at week 4 (odds ratio [OR] 5.7, *P*<.001). Although interleukin (IL)-28B CC genotype was associated with SVR, once the 4-week Peg-IFN/RBV lead-in response was considered, it was no longer a significant predictor.[7]

Preliminary results from a randomized trial of BOC triple therapy using Peg-IFN alfa-2a (rather than alfa-2b) in treatment-experienced patients with entry criteria and treatment arms similar to RESPOND-2 but without an RGT arm, reported SVR rates comparable to RESPOND-2. A total of 64% (86 of 134) BOC-treated patients versus 21% (28 of 67) of controls achieved SVR (P<.001). Similar to the RESPOND-2 study, undetectability of HCV RNA after the 4-week lead-in of Peg-IFN/RBV was associated with higher SVR (71% compared with 39% in those without a lead-in response, P value not given).

Nonrandomized studies
The PROVIDE study is a single-arm, nonrandomized, rollover study of nonresponders to Peg-IFN/RBV from the control arms of the phase 2 and 3 trials for BOC (SPRINT-1, SPRINT-2, RESPOND-2, PEG2a/BOC study). This is an important study as it includes prior null responders. RGT was not used. Interim results of 168 out of 175 enrolled patients revealed an SVR rate in those with previous relapse or partial response of 68% (62 of 91) and 36% for null responders (19 of 47), respectively.[8]

Telaprevir

Randomized controlled trials (TPV)
REALIZE is the pivotal phase 3 trial of 663 patients from 17 international centers comparing triple therapy of TPV 750 mg 3 times daily (every 7–9 hours), Peg-IFN alfa-2a 180 μg/wk and RBV (1000–1200 mg/d) to Peg-IFN/RBV alone in treatment-experienced patients with chronic HCV GT1.[9] The total treatment duration was 48 weeks in all groups (no RGT), but the utility of a 4-week peg-IFN/RBV lead-in was evaluated. Patients were stratified on baseline HCV viral level and previous treatment response (relapse vs partial response vs null response) into

Group 1 (T12PR48) of 12 weeks of TPV, Peg-IFN, and RBV followed by another 36 weeks of Peg-IFN/RBV alone

Group 2 (LI-T12PR48) a 4-week lead-in of placebo/Peg-IFN/RBV followed by 12 weeks of TPV/Peg-IFN/RBV and ending with 32 weeks of Peg-IFN/RBV alone

Group 3 (PR48) receiving placebo/Peg-IFN/RBV for 16 weeks followed by Peg-IFN/RBV for 32 weeks

SVR was assessed 24 weeks after treatment. Noteworthy demographics of the study population are the high proportion of null responders and cirrhotics (25%) and low percentage of African Americans (see **Table 1**). The SVR rates were significantly higher in all arms containing TPV compared with patients who received Peg-IFN/RBV (83% T12PR48 vs 88% LI-T12PR48) versus 24% PR48, (P<.001, see **Fig. 2**). Other predictors of SVR were nonblack race, low baseline HCV RNA, age younger than 40 years, absence of cirrhosis, and statin use (**Table 2**). In the T12PR48 arms, relapse

Table 2		
Stopping rules for PI triple therapy in treatment of GT1 chronic hepatitis C		
Stopping Rules–TPV[a]		
Time point	HCV-RNA result	Action
Week 4 or 12	>1000 IU/mL	Discontinue TPV/Peg-IFN/RBV
Week 24	Detectable	Discontinue Peg-IFN/RBV
Stopping Rules – Boceprevir		
Time point	HCV-RNA result	Action
Week 12	≥100 IU/mL	Discontinue BOC/Peg-IFN/RBV
Week 24	Detectable	Discontinue BOC/Peg-IFN/RBV

[a] Stopping rule used in REALIZE differed from FDA approval stopping rules for TPV.

and virologic failure after treatment discontinuation were more common in those with previous nonresponse (12% and 38%, respectively) compared with prior relapsers (3% and 1%, respectively). Within this group of patients, TPV-resistant variants were common, occurring in 6% (18 of 286) of prior relapsers and 40% (98 of 244) of nonresponders; however, at a median of 9 months of follow-up, 53% (63 of 118) of patients had replacement of resistant viral variants with wild-type virus.[10] The clinical implications of these resistant viral variants are still unclear.

Nonrandomized trials

An open-labeled, nonrandomized, rollover trial was performed among the 117 well-characterized HCV GT1 patients who were nonresponders (relapsers [n = 29], partial responders [n = 29], null responders [n = 51], or prior viral breakthrough, [n = 8]) to the Peg-IFN/RBV control arms of the phase 2 trials for TPV (PROVE-1, PROVE-2, PROVE-3).[11] In this rollover trial, TPV 750 mg 3 times daily (7–9 hours) was administered with Peg-IFN alfa-2a 180 μg/wk and weight-based RBV (1000–1200 mg/d) as RGT in those with prior relapse, viral breakthrough, or partial response.[11] Patients with undetectable HCV RNA at weeks 4 and 12 completed another 12 weeks of Peg-IFN/RBV alone for a total of 24 weeks; those who did not attain these virologic benchmarks completed an additional 36 weeks of Peg-IFN/RBV for a total of 48 weeks of treatment. Null responders were initially intended to receive RGT for a total of 24 weeks; however, a protocol revision based on phase 2 study results extended treatment duration in null responders to a total of 48 weeks therapy (36 weeks of Peg-IFN/RBV after 12 weeks of TPV triple therapy). The overall SVR rate was 57%, with the highest rates among those with previous relapse (97%), followed by viral breakthrough (75%), partial response (55%), and null response (37%).[11]

Importance of cirrhosis

Regardless of the PI used, SVR rates are lower among those with advanced fibrosis (bridging fibrosis and cirrhosis) compared with those with less severe stages of fibrosis.[6,8,9,11,12] Overall, the number of patients with cirrhosis included in prior studies of PI triple therapy was limited, especially among BOC-treated patients.[6,8,9,11,12] Consequently, the estimates of SVR among patients with cirrhosis are less precise than with noncirrhotic patients. Among TPV-treated patients, SVR rates are 34% and 14% for partial and null responders with cirrhosis, respectively, compared with 67% and 40% in noncirrhotic patients.[9] Among BOC-treated partial responders and relapsers, SVR rates are 59% in cirrhotic patients and 65% in noncirrhotic patients (as noted previously, null responders were not included in this trial).[6] The reduced rate of SVR was partially overcome by extending treatment duration. For example, among partial responders and relapsers with cirrhosis re-treated with BOC triple therapy, SVR rates were 35% for RGT and 77% for 48 weeks of treatment.[13] Thus, all treatment-experienced patients with cirrhosis are recommended to have treatment for 48 weeks regardless of their on-treatment virologic response. Additionally, patients with cirrhosis require regular surveillance for hepatocellular carcinoma (HCC)[14] and esophageal varices.[15]

Importance of Peg-IFN and RBV lead-in As highlighted, prior response history influences the likelihood of responding to PI triple therapy. For those whose prior on-treatment response to Peg-IFN/RBV is unknown, the 4-week lead-in period of Peg-IFN/RBV before start of triple therapy provides important information on IFN responsiveness. For example, the virologic response during the lead-in period of the REALIZE trial with TPV, and all the BOC trials, was shown to be an important predictor of SVR. In RESPOND-2 (BOC-triple therapy), a <1 log IU/mL decline in

HCV RNA during the first 4 weeks of treatment was associated with SVR rates of 33% to 34% compared with SVR rates of 75% to 79% in those with at least a 1 log IU/mL decline (OR = 5.2, P<.001).[7] Further, among those with poor IFN responsiveness (<1 log HCV RNA decline during 4-week lead-in), the magnitude of the HCV viral load decline at week 8 of treatment (after 4 weeks of BOC/Peg-IFN/RBV) was highly predictive of non-SVR. In this group, no patient with a less than 3 log decline in HCV RNA at week 8 achieved SVR, suggesting this could be used as a treatment stopping rule.[16] In contrast, in patients with an initial poor response during lead-in but who achieved an undetectable HCV RNA at week 8, the likelihood of SVR was 91%. In the REALIZE study (TPV-triple therapy), a drop of at least 1 log in viral load after 4 weeks of Peg-IFN/RBV was associated with increased SVR rates with subsequent TPV triple therapy compared with those who did not, especially among prior null responders (15% vs 59%). No difference was observed in the partial responders (54% vs 56%), and the differences in SVR among prior relapsers with at least a 1 log drop versus less than 1log drop in viral load was 88% versus 62%.[17] Therefore, in patients whose previous response to Peg-IFN-RBV is unknown, a 4-week lead-in of Peg-IFN/RBV may be a very useful way to identify patients more likely to achieve SVR to PI triple therapy (see section titled "Treatment of patients with unknown prior response").

PRACTICAL APPROACH TO PATIENT WITH PRIOR RELAPSE WITH PEG-IFN AND RBV

Patients with previous relapse to Peg-IFN/RBV are excellent candidates for re-treatment using PI triple therapy with either TPV or BOC, with SVR rates of 83% to 88% and 69% to 75% respectively **Fig. 3**.[6,9] Similarities in the TPV and BOC triple therapy regimens include the use of RGT for noncirrhotic patients and fixed 48 weeks therapy for cirrhotic patients. Differences between the PI treatment regimens include use of lead-in (BOC only) and duration of treatment with RGT (24 weeks TPV, 36 weeks BOC). RGT and stopping rules are the same as in treatment-naïve patients (see **Table 2**).

Ability to Use RGT

An RGT approach can be used for noncirrhotic patients with a history of previous relapse.

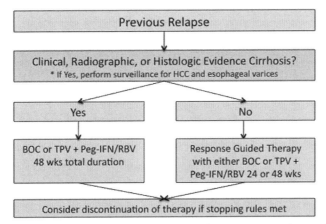

Fig. 3. Suggested treatment for patients with prior relapse to Peg-IFN/RBV. *Abbreviations:* BOC, boceprevir; HCC, hepatocellular carcinoma; TPV, telaprevir.

Patients who achieve nondetectable levels of HCV RNA at weeks 4 through 12 on TPV-containing triple therapy are eligible for a treatment duration that is identical to that of treatment-naïve patients (ie, 24 weeks). Although RGT was not evaluated in the REALIZE trial, the recommendation for RGT is based on the noninferiority of RGT versus 48 weeks therapy in treatment-naïve patients treated with TPV and the observation that 76% of relapsers in REALIZE (218 of 286 patients) achieved an extended rapid virologic response (eRVR, undetectable HCV RNA at weeks 4 and 12), and of those, 95% (208 of 218 patients) achieved an SVR.[9] In addition, in an earlier smaller dose-finding study with TPV-containing triple therapy, 78% (52 of 67) of prior relapsers achieved undetectable HCV RNA at weeks 4 through 12, and of these 94% (49 of 52 patients) achieved an SVR with 24 weeks treatment.[18] The lead-in arm of 4 weeks of Peg-IFN/RBV was not found to provide any benefit in relapsers and is not recommended with TPV triple therapy.[9]

If BOC triple therapy is used, patients who are HCV RNA-negative at weeks 8 to 24 are eligible to have a shorter duration of treatment (ie, 36 weeks), whereas as those failing to achieve HCV RNA negativity by week 8 of treatment require an additional 12 weeks of Peg-IFN/RBV (total 48 weeks). In the RESPOND-2 study, 49% of combined relapser/partial responders were HCV RNA negative at week 8 of combination therapy. The SVR rates between the RGT and 48-week arms were not significantly different (ie, 68.6% and 74.8%, respectively).[6]

Considerations if Cirrhosis is Present

RGT is not recommended for relapsers with cirrhosis, although the data to support this recommendation are relatively limited. In relapsers with cirrhosis treated with BOC triple therapy, SVR rates were 77% (17 of 22 patients) with 48 weeks treatment compared with 35% (6 of 17 patients) with RGT.[6] SVR rates among relapsers with cirrhosis treated with RGT versus 48 weeks TPV triple therapy are not available. However, among treatment-naïve patients with cirrhosis treated with TPV triple therapy, in those patients with undetectable HCV RNA at week 4 (through week 12) who received 48 weeks of therapy a higher SVR rate (91%, 11/12) was found than than in those who received 24 weeks of therapy (67%, 12 of 18 patients).[19]

APPROACH TO THE PATIENT WITH PRIOR PARTIAL RESPONSE TO PEG-IFN AND RBV

Patients with previous partial response to Peg-IFN/RBV are reasonable candidates for PI triple therapy with SVR rates of 54% to 59% and 40% to 52% with TPV triple therapy and BOC triple therapy, respectively (**Fig. 4**; see **Fig. 1**).[6,9] However, host and viral factors influence these SVR rates and should be taken into consideration when making the decision to treat.

Ability to Use RGT

This is only a potential option with BOC triple therapy. Recommendations for use of RGT with BOC triple therapy differ in the United States versus Europe (US Food and Drug Administration [FDA] vs European Medicines Agency [EMA]). The FDA approved a BOC triple therapy regimen in partial responders that is the same as in relapsers (ie, RGT); patients with undetectable HCV RNA at weeks 8 through 24 of treatment are eligible for a total treatment duration of 36 weeks, while those who do not achieve this early virologic response need an additional 12 weeks of Peg-IFN/RBV (48 weeks total treatment). However, the EMA did not approve RGT for partial responders; thus, a 48-week treatment duration is recommended. Of note, the difference in SVR rates with BOC triple therapy among partial responders treated with RGT

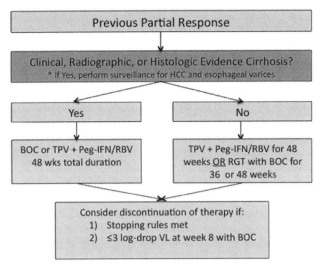

Fig. 4. Suggested treatment of patients with prior partial response to Peg-IFN/RBV. *Abbreviations:* BOC, boceprevir; HCC, hepatocellular carcinoma; RGT, response-guided therapy; TPV, telaprevir.

versus 48 weeks of therapy is not actually known, as only combined relapser/partial responder data are available.

Data on partial responders treated with TPV triple therapy using an RGT approach versus a fixed 48 weeks of therapy are unavailable. In the absence of such data, the recommended treatment duration is 48 weeks, with TPR/Peg-IFN/RBV given for 12 weeks of followed by Peg-IFN/RBV for 36 weeks, in those meeting on-treatment response endpoints (see **Table 2**).

Considerations if Cirrhosis is Present

Partial responders with cirrhosis have a lower rate of a sustained response than non-cirrhotic patients, regardless of the PI triple therapy used. All cirrhotic patients with a history of a partial response should be treated for 48 weeks, regardless of early virologic responses. In TPV-treated patients with partial response, SVR was attained in 72% (34 of 47) of those with minimal fibrosis (F 0–2) versus 34% (11 of 32) in those with cirrhosis.[9] For BOC triple therapy, the SVR rates for partial responders and relapsers combined were 44% among patients with F3/4 fibrosis versus 68% among those with less fibrosis.[6] Overall, the limited number of prior partial responders with cirrhosis studied hinders the precision of the available estimates of SVR, but it appears that an approximately 40% SVR rate can be anticipated in partial responders with cirrhosis treated with triple therapy.[6,9]

APPROACH TO THE PATIENT WITH PRIOR NULL RESPONSE TO PEG-IFN AND RBV

Rates of SVR in null responders are higher with PI triple therapy compared Peg-IFN/RBV, but are still suboptimal, with SVR rates of 29% to 37% with TPV and 36% with BOC **Fig. 5**.[8,9,12] Thus, many of these patients may be better served by deferring retreatment until more efficacious therapies are available. However, the decision to defer treatment must be tempered by consideration of disease- and patient-specific

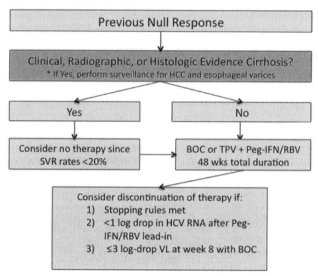

Fig. 5. Suggested treatment of patients with prior null response to Peg-IFN/RBV. Abbreviations: BOC, boceprevir; HCC, hepatocellular carcinoma; TPV, telaprevir; VL, viral load.

factors influencing both likelihood of SVR and the risk of future complications in the absence of re-treatment.

Ability to Use RGT

RGT is not recommended for any patient with a prior null response regardless of the PI being considered due to the lower SVR rates with shorter therapy.

Considerations if Cirrhosis is Present

Since all null responders are treated for 48 weeks, the presence of cirrhosis in null responders does not affect the treatment duration as in other subgroups. However, cirrhosis has important implications for the expected response to treatment. In null responders with underlying cirrhosis treated with TPV triple therapy, the SVR rates are 14%.[9] Specific information on the SVR rates in cirrhotic null responders treated with BOC triple therapy are lacking (only 4% of the patients included in PROVIDE study), but SVR rates are unlikely to be higher. Thus, the benefits versus risks of PI triple therapy should be weighed carefully for cirrhotic patients with prior null response. In these difficult-to-cure patients, a lead-in of Peg-IFN/RBV may help identify those with highest likelihood of SVR. For example, in the REALIZE study (TPV-triple therapy), null responders (all stages of disease) with at least a 1 log decline in HCV RNA after lead-in had an SVR rate of 59% versus 15% in those without a decline of HCV RNA of a least 1log during lead-in.[20]

TREATMENT OF PATIENTS WITH UNKNOWN PRIOR RESPONSE

A proportion of patients presenting for consideration of antiviral treatment lack treatment records documenting the virologic response during prior treatment. The absence of this information is limiting in 2 principle ways. First, because SVR rates are highly influenced by prior response status, the discussion with the patient about expected SVR rates with PI triple therapy retreatment are more difficult. Second, the duration of treatment will be unknown. The latter is less an issue if the patient has cirrhosis, as all these patients are treated for 48 weeks. For noncirrhotic patients, RGT is an option for relapsers and BOC-treated partial responders but not other groups.

Three different approaches to this scenario can be considered:

1. Treat all patients as if they are null responders. With this approach, the patient receives 48 weeks of treatment, independent of on-treatment virologic responses. This approach maximizes the likelihood of SVR but will result in overtreatment of a proportion of patients (ie, prior relapsers).
2. Use the Peg-IFN/RBV lead-in to estimate prior response status before initiation of PI (TPV or BOC) therapy. While the classic definition of partial and null response requires 12 weeks of treatment, the response to 4 weeks of Peg-IFN/RBV can yield useful information. In RESPOND-2 (BOC-triple therapy), patients who achieved at least a 1 log drop in HCV RNA after a 4-week lead-in had SVR rates of 73% and 79% with or without RGT, respectively.[16] Similarly, SVR rates were higher in individuals treated with TPV in REALIZE if the week-4 HCV RNA dropped by at least 1 log IU/mL.[20] With this approach, patients with poor IFN-response will receive 48 weeks treatment, and those with good IFN-response may be considered for RGT. This approach reduces the number of patients who are unnecessarily treated for 48 weeks but may undertreat some patients.
3. Use the response at week 4 or 8 of treatment to determine treatment duration. The achievement of undetectable HCV RNA levels by week 4 of TPV triple therapy and week 8 of BOC triple therapy is highly predictive of SVR. Thus, one could consider using RGT for those who achieve undetectability at this early time point and 48 weeks therapy for those who do not. Like the previous strategy, this approach reduces the number of patients who are treated for longer than necessary but may undertreat some patients.

TREAT NOW OR WAIT FOR BETTER THERAPIES?

Attaining sustained clearance of HCV is the goal of treatment. Achievement of SVR has been shown to halt (and in some cases reverse) fibrosis progression and decrease the risk of hepatic decompensation, need for liver transplantation, development of hepatocellular carcinoma, and overall mortality.[21] PI triple therapy with BOC and TVR has substantially improved the chances for SVR, but it is now known that there are many other HCV drugs in the development pipeline. Additionally, more efficacious and better-tolerated therapies are expected in the future. Thus, patients and providers need to decide whether to undertake treatment now versus await future new drug therapies.

The factors to consider include:

1. Anticipated SVR rates. As highlighted, relapsers have a high likelihood of SVR with TPV triple therapy or BOC triple therapy, and the majority will require only 24 to 28 weeks of therapy. Thus, this subgroup is well suited for treatment with current PI triple therapy. Other favorable groups in terms of higher rates of SVR include those with low fibrosis score, low (<800,000 IU/mL) HCV viral load, and favorable host factors, including IL-28B genotype.[22]
2. Anticipated tolerability of therapy. Patients who previously tolerated Peg-IFN/RBV therapy and those with a limited number of comorbidities are generally good candidates for consideration for retreatment with PI triple therapy. Patients who had difficulty tolerating Peg-IFN/RBV and needed drug interruption or discontinuation due to adverse effects may be poor candidates for re-treatment with PI triple therapy.

3. Risk of disease progression while awaiting new therapies. Any treatment-experienced patient with advanced fibrosis or underlying cirrhosis (F3/F4) should more strongly consider BOC triple therapy or TPV triple therapy given the potential benefits of obtaining SVR and the potential for further hepatic damage while awaiting newer drugs. The potential treatment benefits are particularly clear for relapsers and partial responders. However, the decision to treat the previous null responder is more difficult, since the demonstrated SVR rates are less than 20%. If treatment is deferred, these patients need to be followed closely for evidence of progression while awaiting other treatment options.

REFERENCES

1. Manns MP, McHutchison JG, Gordon SC, et al. Peginterferon alfa-2b plus ribavirin compared with interferon alfa-2b plus ribavirin for initial treatment of chronic hepatitis C: a randomised trial. Lancet 2001;358(9286):958–65.
2. Jensen DM, Marcellin P, Freilich B, et al. Re-treatment of patients with chronic hepatitis C who do not respond to peginterferon-alpha2b: a randomized trial. Ann Intern Med 2009;150(8):528–40.
3. Poynard T, Colombo M, Bruix J, et al. Peginterferon alfa-2b and ribavirin: effective in patients with hepatitis C who failed interferon alfa/ribavirin therapy. Gastroenterology 2009;136(5):1618–1628.e2.
4. Sherman M, Yoshida EM, Deschenes M, et al. Peginterferon alfa-2a (40KD) plus ribavirin in chronic hepatitis C patients who failed previous interferon therapy. Gut 2006;55(11):1631–8.
5. Taliani G, Gemignani G, Ferrari C, et al. Pegylated interferon alfa-2b plus ribavirin in the retreatment of interferon–ribavirin nonresponder patients. Gastroenterology 2006;130(4):1098–106.
6. Bacon BR, Gordon SC, Lawitz E, et al. Boceprevir for previously treated chronic HCV genotype 1 infection. N Engl J Med 2011;364(13):1207–17.
7. Zeuzem S, Vierling JM, Esteban R, et al. Predictors of sustained virologic response among genotype 1 previous non-responders and relapsers to peginterferon/ribavirin when re-treated with boceprevir plus peginterferon alpha-2b/ribavirin (abstract #484). Hepatology 2011;54(Suppl 1):S198–9.
8. Bronowicki JP, Davis M, Flamm S, et al. Sustained virologic response (SVR) in prior PegInterferon/ribavirin (PR) treatment failures after retreatment with boceprevir (BOC) + PR: the PROVIDE Study Interim Results (abstract #11). Hepatology 2012;56(Suppl 2):S5.
9. Zeuzem S, Andreone P, Pol S, et al. Telaprevir for retreatment of HCV infection. N Engl J Med 2011;364(25):2417–28.
10. Kieffer TL, De Meyer S, Bartels DJ, et al. Hepatitis C viral evolution in genotype 1 treatment-naive and treatment-experienced patients receiving telaprevir-based therapy in clinical trials. PLoS One 2012;7(4):e34372.
11. Muir AJ, Poordad FF, McHutchison JG, et al. Retreatment with telaprevir combination therapy in hepatitis C patients with well-characterized prior treatment response. Hepatology 2011;54(5):1538–46.
12. Flamm S, Lawitz E, Jacobson I, et al. High sustained virologic response (SVR) among genotype 1 previous non-responders and relapsers to peginterferon/ribavirin when re-treated with boceprevir (BOC) plus peginterferon alfa-2a/ribavirin (abstract #1366). Hepatology 2011;54(Suppl 1):S541–2.
13. Victrelis (package insert). Merck & Co., Inc., Whitehouse Station, NJ.

14. Bruix J, Sherman M, American Association for the Study of Liver Diseases. Management of hepatocellular carcinoma: an update. Hepatology 2011;53(3):1020–2.
15. Garcia-Tsao G, Sanyal AJ, Grace ND, et al, Practice Guidelines Committee of the American Association for the Study of Liver Diseases, Practice Parameters Committee of the American College of Gastroenterology. Prevention and management of gastroesophageal varices and variceal hemorrhage in cirrhosis. Hepatology 2007;46(3):922–38.
16. Bacon BR, Bruno S, Schiff E, et al. Predictors of sustained virologic response among poor interferon responders when boceprevir is added to peginterferon alpha-2b/ribavirin (abstract #33). AASLD 2011.
17. Foster GR, Zeuzem S, Andreone P, et al. Subanalyses of the telaprevir lead-in arm in the REALIZE study: response at week 4 is not a substitute for prior null response categorization. J Hepatol 2011;54(Suppl 1):S3.
18. Incivek (package insert). Vertex Pharmaceuticals Incorporated, Cambridge, MA.
19. Sherman KE, Flamm SL, Afdhal NH, et al. Response-guided telaprevir combination treatment for hepatitis C virus infection. N Engl J Med 2011;365(11):1014–24.
20. Foster GR, Zeuzem P, Pol S, et al. Subanalyses of the telaprevir lead-in arm in the REALIZE Study: Response at week 4 is not a substitute for prior null response categorization. Hepatology 2011;54(Suppl 1):S3–4.
21. Singal AG, Volk ML, Jensen D, et al. A sustained viral response is associated with reduced liver-related morbidity and mortality in patients with hepatitis C virus. Clin Gastroenterol Hepatol 2010;8(3):280–8.
22. Pacanowski M, Amur A, Zineh I. New genetic discoveries and treatment for hepatitis C. JAMA 2012;307(18):1921–2.

Managing Adverse Effects of Interferon-Alfa and Ribavirin in Combination Therapy for HCV

Jihad Slim, MD*, Muhammad Shoaib Afridi, MD

KEYWORDS

- Interferon-alfa • Ribavirin • Hepatitis C virus • Adverse effects

KEY POINTS

- The most common side effects of interferon-alfa therapy are flulike symptoms, which are controlled with nonsteroidal anti-inflammatory drugs and abate with time. Other common symptoms include fatigue, loss of appetite, and weight loss.
- Depression is generally effectively treated with selective serotonin reuptake inhibitors; however, if major depressive symptoms are not recognized and treated, patients treated with interferon-alfa are at risk for suicide.
- The most common cause of anemia during HCV therapy is a dose-dependent hemolysis secondary to ribavirin, best managed by dose reduction.
- Autoimmune diseases can be exacerbated by interferon-alfa, and usually resolve after cessation of therapy.
- Patients with diabetic or hypertensive retinopathy should be regularly followed by an ophthalmologist while on therapy with interferon-alfa.
- Patients should be counseled regarding ribavirin's teratogenic effects, which can occur up to 6 months after treatment is discontinued because of its long half-life.

INTRODUCTION

This article focuses on the adverse effects (AEs) of hepatitis C therapy, which includes pegylated interferon (IFN) alfa-2a or -2b with ribavirin (RBV). The AEs of the newer direct-acting antiviral agents are not discussed, unless they produce side effects in conjunction with IFN and RBV therapy. To fully understand the management of the spectrum of AEs in Chronic Active Hepatitis C (CAH-C) therapy, the pathophysiology of IFN and RBV on a molecular level should be understood, along with indications for modification of the treatment regimen. The hepatitis C virus (HCV) provider should

St. Michaels Medical Center, 111 Central Avenue, Newark, NJ 07102, USA
* Corresponding author.
E-mail address: jsmdsmmc@gmail.com

Infect Dis Clin N Am 26 (2012) 917–929
http://dx.doi.org/10.1016/j.idc.2012.08.006
0891-5520/12/$ – see front matter © 2012 Elsevier Inc. All rights reserved.

remain cognizant of the various organ systems that can be affected, which AEs should be addressed with the help of an expert, and the presentation of symptoms as they occur throughout the course of therapy. A systems-based approach should help to characterize the nature of the AEs that patients experience, and also to determine when patients should be further investigated by a consultant.

PATHOPHYSIOLOGY OF IFN-ALFA

IFNs communicate between cells to trigger the protective defenses of the immune system when presented with biochemical injury, whether from viruses, bacteria, or tumor cells. IFN-alfa is a natural cytokine whose receptors are ubiquitous in the body, and once bound to the cell surface receptor, IFN activates tyrosine kinases. This tyrosine kinase pathway leads to the production of several IFN-stimulated enzymes, such as $2'$-$5'$-oligoadenylate synthetase and β_2 microglobulin.[1] These, and possibly other IFN-stimulated enzymes, are thought to be responsible for the range of pleiotropic effects of IFN-alfa, which are antiviral, antiproliferative, and immunomodulatory. IFNs also play a key role in cellular differentiation; upregulation of major histocompatibility antigen expression (HLA class I); and cytokine induction. Pegylation of the IFN chemical has lengthened the half-life of IFN alfa-2a and IFN alfa-2b is prolonged by the process of pegylation, thus making it more efficacious but with an increase in the rate of side effects.[2]

PATHOPHYSIOLOGY OF RBV

RBV monotherapy is associated with improvement in aminotransferases, but has only a modest antiviral effect of approximately one-half log. However, in the 1990s, the combination of standard thrice weekly IFN with RBV substantially improved sustained virologic response (SVR) rates over IFN monotherapy.[3] The exact mechanism of action for RBV is not well known, but its side effect profile has been well characterized. RBV causes a dose-dependent hemolytic anemia that seems to be related to the accumulation of RBV in the erythrocyte; this leads to reduction in intracellular ATP levels, subsequently impairing glutathione levels and permitting oxidative lysis of erythrocytes.[4] The other side effect of concern is teratogenicity.

Most AEs can be managed appropriately with dose reductions. However, special attention must be given to preserve efficacy of the treatment while avoiding serious medication effects. Balancing the amount of exposure to IFN and RBV to achieve SVR with the AEs is an important aspect of treating CAH-C with dual antiviral therapy, particularly patients with genotype 1 infection.[5,6] However, when using triple therapy including an HCV protease inhibitor, dose reductions do not seem to have a negative effect on overall virologic outcome in patients with genotype 1 infection.

Despite the array of side effects experienced with combination therapy, the rate of discontinuation secondary to AEs in most clinical trials nears 10%. A systems-based review of the management of side effects allows the HCV provider to approach CAH-C therapy with detail to drug reduction, and treatment withdrawal with emphasis on pathophysiology of the symptoms when pertinent, especially at the start of therapy.

SYSTEMIC COMPLICATIONS

Most patients treated with IFN and RBV report several systemic complaints that can be subdivided into three categories: (1) flulike symptoms, (2) fatigue, and (3) weight loss (**Table 1**).

Table 1
Commonly encountered adverse effects and their management

Adverse Effect	Management
Flulike symptoms	Nonsteroidal anti-inflammatory drugs postinjection
	Nonsteroidal anti-inflammatory drug prophylaxis if symptoms severe
Depression	Selective serotonin reuptake inhibitors
Hypothyroidism	Hormone replacement, monitor thyroid-stimulating hormone every 4 wks
Hyperthyroidism	Endocrine consultation
Dry skin, pruritus	Topical antipruritics, good hydration
	Systemic antihistamines
Alopecia	Supportive care, and reassurance

Flulike Symptoms

Flulike symptoms consisting of fever, chills, arthralgias, myalgias, rigors, headache, fatigue, and weakness are the most frequent side effects reported by patients receiving IFN. These symptoms usually start a few hours after the injection, and last for 24 to 48 hours.[2,3] After the first few injections symptoms are more severe, but tend to abate after 5 to 6 weeks on therapy.[5] IFN-induced release of cytokines, such as tumor necrosis factor-α, interleukin-1, and interleukin-6, are most likely responsible for the host of symptoms that occur.[7]

Patients can modify the effect of the symptoms on their lifestyle if they schedule the injection, treat with anti-inflammatory medications, and even use acetaminophen and over-the-counter nonsteroidal anti-inflammatory drugs (NSAIDs) prophylactically if they cannot tolerate the AEs. If patients take their injection at night, and before the days of the week when they have a light schedule, they can prevent AEs from altering their daily activities. Patients with flulike symptoms rarely have to stop treatment or reduce their IFN dose.

Fatigue

Up to two-thirds of patients complain of fatigue, which is a common side effect of IFN therapy. However, it is important that the clinician distinguish fatigue from severe anemia or depression or other metabolic disorders (eg, hypothyroidism).[3]

During patient visits, the provider must be cognizant of hemoglobin levels, mood stability, and medication adherence, all possible indicators of fatigue. A large drop in hemoglobin level over a short period of time causes more fatigue than a similar change of hemoglobin levels over a longer period of time. Larger drops of hemoglobin may also precipitate shortness of breath.

In addition to hemoglobin values, thyroid laboratory markers should be screened and followed throughout therapy. IFN use may lead to either hypothyroidism, which can be treated with hormone replacement, or hyperthyroidism, which often requires expert medical management.

The clinician should always assess the patient for depression at baseline and at each subsequent clinic visit with a depression scale questionnaire, in addition to complaints of insomnia, headaches, and mood changes. Patients with mild depression at baseline may better cope with HCV therapy if given an antidepressant or mood stabilizer. Patients who develop severe depression should be discontinued off HCV therapy, regardless of whether they are attaining a virologic response, because suicide has been reported on combination therapy.

Although rare, neuropathy, myopathy, and cardiomyopathy have all been described during therapy with IFN and in the appropriate clinical setting warrant evaluation.[8]

Weight Loss

Weight loss is seen mainly with IFN use, and is reported more frequently in patients coinfected with HIV.[9] Weight loss stems from poor oral intake secondary to nausea, which is reported in at least a third of patients; hyperthyroidism secondary to thyroiditis; anorexia with or without depression; and direct effect of cytokines on myocytes.[3] It rarely leads to treatment discontinuation, and is managed depending on the underlying cause.

Weight loss occurs less frequently with the newer protease inhibitor combinations with boceprevir and telaprevir, most likely because food is required with both agents.

HEMATOLOGIC COMPLICATIONS

Anemia, thrombocytopenia (TCP), and neutropenia are the primary AEs to occur during IFN-RBV therapy and can exacerbate pre-existing conditions for which patients should be screened. Patients with HCV may have other conditions that require treatment with medications (eg, proton-pump inhibitors or H_2 blockers causing idiopathic thrombocytopenic purpura, or zidovudine causing anemia) that could cause hematologic toxicities. A multifaceted approach is required to manage the cytopenia-related AEs with pretreatment screening, cardiac and hematologic consultations when necessary, frequent laboratory monitoring, and dose reductions to ensure the safety of the patient while trying to maintain as much drug exposure as possible.

Anemia

The most frequent hematologic AE that results in dose reduction or discontinuation of RBV and sometimes IFN is anemia.[8] At baseline, a complete assessment of risk factors for anemia and coronary artery disease (CAD) should be performed and high-risk patients referred to a cardiologist for an abnormal stress test and clearance for therapy. Regular complete blood count observation is crucial to prevent myocardial injury in patients with underlying CAD. Lower hemoglobin levels increase cardiac demand and may stress the heart resulting in an acute myocardial infarction in patients with underlying CAD (**Table 2**). The risk for acute myocardial infarction increases substantially with acute drops in hemoglobin; however, hemoglobin concentrations must still be followed frequently even among patients with slow declines in hemoglobin. Frequent monitoring is especially important if telaprevir or boceprevir are added to IFN-RBV therapy, because these HCV protease inhibitors are associated with a significant additional decline in hemoglobin concentrations.

Anemia can have multiples causes and a basic anemia work-up is essential in the patient with pre-existing anemia. Baseline tests should be performed, including iron,

Table 2	
The most dangerous adverse effects and their management	
Adverse Effect	**Management**
Suicidal ideation	Stop IFN
Acute myocardial infarction	Stop treatment
Ischemic colitis	Colonoscopy and CT scan, stop IFN
Interstitial pneumonitis	High-resolution scan, DLCO, stop IFN

Abbreviation: DLCO, Carbon monoxide diffusing capacity.

total iron binding capacity, ferritin, reticulocyte count, conjugated bilirubin, lactate dehydrogenase, haptoglobin, vitamin B_{12}, folate, and complete blood count. Treatment of the underlying cause of anemia is advised before initiation of HCV therapy. Further investigation (eg, colonoscopy) is sometimes needed when a diagnosis is not apparent initially, such as iron-deficiency anemia in a male patient.

RBV should be used very cautiously in patients with various comorbidities, such as renal insufficiency; dose reductions are based on the degree of renal disease. Treatment with RBV also requires close supervision in patients with cirrhosis who may develop severe anemia. RBV is contraindicated in patients with pre-existing hemoglobinopathies.[10] In the past, the risk of RBV-associated anemia was markedly higher among patients infected with HIV who were treated with zidovudine, which used to be a first-line agent for the treatment of HIV but is uncommonly used today.

RBV dose can usually be adjusted or held for a limited time period (**Table 3**). In light of the long half-life of the drug (~12 days in serum and ~40 days in erythrocytes), holding the dose until the hemoglobin level is stable is prudent, especially in patients with underlying stable CAD. This RBV dose-reduction strategy does not seem to decrease SVR rates in patients receiving telaprevir in conjunction with IFN-RBV combination therapy. Patients with inosine triphosphatase activity deficiency are less likely to develop anemia secondary to RBV, but testing for this genetic polymorphism is not routinely done.[11]

If the anemia is found to be nonhemolytic, with low reticulocyte count, normal lactate dehydrogenase, and haptoglobin level, then IFN is most likely inducing bone marrow suppression, usually accompanied with TCP and neutropenia.[12]

Before the use of telaprevir and boceprevir, many clinicians used erythrocyte growth factors, such as erythropoietin, early in therapy. Although erythropoietin was associated with an improved quality of life, it was not clear that erythropoietin was associated with better virologic response rates. In clinical practice, erythropoietin has been replaced for the most part by RBV dose reduction with close monitoring of the hemoglobin level.[13] Erythropoietin use is not without its own complications and may be considered when the hemoglobin level drops lower than 10 g/dL, but should be held if the level recovers higher than 10 g/dL to prevent a cerebrovascular accident. A recent clinical trial in patients taking boceprevir/PEG/RBV demonstrated that overall SVR rates were comparable whether the patient was assigned to erythropoietin or RBV dose reduction (Sulkowski EASL).

Thrombocytopenia

TCP is a well-known side effect of IFN and the risk of TCP increases with use of the HCV protease inhibitors. Protease inhibitors likely cause suppression of transcription factors regulating late-stage megakaryopoiesis; this complication is managed mainly

Table 3
Ribavirin dose modification for anemia

Laboratory Values	Reduce RBV Dose to 600 mg/day If:	Discontinue RBV If:
Hemoglobin in patients with no cardiac disease	<10 g/dL	<8.5 g/dL
Hemoglobin in patients with history of stable cardiac disease	≥2 g/dL decrease in hemoglobin during any 4-wk period treatment	<12 g/dL despite 4 wks at reduced dose

with IFN dose reduction (**Table 4**).[14,15] The patient's medication list should also be reviewed to determine if any drug could be causing TCP. In the setting of TCP, hemolysis secondary to RBV can lead to a compensatory thrombocytosis, which can lessen the severity of the TCP.

Patients with advanced-stage liver fibrosis and pre-existing hypersplenism are at highest risk to experience further worsening of their baseline TCP. However, TCP uncommonly leads to drug discontinuation (see **Table 4**). If low platelets persist, the IFN package insert recommends drug discontinuation lower than 50,000/mm^3. Eltrombopag, an oral agonist of the thrombopoietin receptor, is currently being evaluated for the treatment of TCP, but cannot be recommended for routine use at present because preliminary data suggest an increased risk of portal vein thrombosis.[16]

Neutropenia

Pegylated IFN can lead to neutropenia, which can usually be managed with dose modification or growth factors (**Table 5**). In clinical practice the dosage of IFN is often maintained and physicians favor the use of granulocyte colony–stimulating factor if absolute neutrophil count is persistently lower than 500, despite the lack of supporting evidence. Its use for the most part is well tolerated, but can cause bone pain, myalgias, and fever, and it is expensive.

Infectious complications of IFN therapy are uncommon and seem to be independent of the incidence and extent of decrease in the absolute neutrophil count.[17]

PSYCHIATRIC COMPLICATIONS

Psychiatric effects of HCV therapy are relatively preventable through aggressive symptom monitoring and management, frequent visits to assess clinical improvement, the use of selective serotonin reuptake inhibitors, and IFN dose reduction when appropriate, using expert consultation for complex patients (**Table 6**).

Initially, a psychiatric evaluation using a depression scale questionnaire highlights any potential problems and alerts the provider to engage the help of a psychiatrist early in the course of therapy, especially if the patient is at high risk for depression. Risk factors for uncontrolled depression, such as relapse of drug addiction, aggressive behavior, psychoses, hallucinations, bipolar disorders, and mania, are very likely to need psychiatric intervention and monitoring to ensure the patient's safety. Psychiatric AEs can be recognized early and treated aggressively to avoid one of the most feared complications of therapy: suicide.[18,19]

Fatigue that is not well explained may lead to decreased medication adherence possibly because of depression; thus, treatment with selective serotonin reuptake inhibitors is recommended. Clinical evidence points toward citalopram as the most experienced selective serotonin reuptake inhibitor in this setting; however, it can take a few weeks before optimal clinical efficacy is reached.[20]

In addition to fatigue, the HCV provider may observe symptoms that could be related to depression, cognitive impairment, or even psychosis, such as sleep

Table 4			
Pegylated interferon dose modification for thrombocytopenia			
Type of Pegylated Interferon	**Platelets <80,000/L**	**Platelets <50,000/L**	**Platelets <25,000/L**
Alfa-2a	—	Reduce dose by 50%	Discontinue
Alfa-2b	Reduce dose by 50%	Discontinue	Discontinue

Table 5
Pegylated interferon dose modification for neutropenia

Type of Pegylated Interferon	ANC <750 Cells/mm^3	ANC <500 Cells/mm^3
Alfa-2a	Reduce to 135 μg/wk	Discontinue
Alfa-2b	Reduce dose by 50%	Discontinue

disturbance, irritability, difficulty concentrating, and decreased memory. With the onset of these symptoms, it is imperative for the provider to intervene pharmacologically to help patients adhere to therapy.[21] It is important to monitor patients closely at Weeks 2 and 4 of therapy to assess for side effects and even more frequently if symptomatic; otherwise, asymptomatic patients can be scheduled to return every 4 weeks.

In the present era of direct-acting antiviral agents use for genotype 1, reducing the IFN dose temporarily until moderate symptoms resolve may be a good strategy until the drug intervention has proved effective. Patients who were initially started on antidepressant therapy before HCV therapy should taper off slowly during the course of few weeks to avoid withdrawal symptoms.

OPHTHALMOLOGIC COMPLICATIONS

Patients with pre-existing eye disease may be at a higher predisposed risk for IFN-related ocular complications; their care should be coordinated closely with the ophthalmologist. Retinal artery necrosis, vein thrombosis, optic neuritis, papilledema, retinal hemorrhages, and cotton-wool spots are all complications of IFN therapy, of which the latter two are more frequent.[22] Retinal hemorrhages and cotton-wool spots are more prevalent in patients with pre-existing diabetic retinopathy.

The Federal Drug Advisory board recommends all patients undergoing IFN therapy have a baseline retinal examination; those with pre-existing ophthalmologic disorders (eg, diabetic or hypertensive retinopathy) should receive periodic ophthalmologic examinations during therapy.

Patients who complain of blurry vision, loss of vision, or greying of the visual field should receive a prompt and complete eye examination. The decision to stop IFN should be made in coordination with the ophthalmologist, considering the ocular findings, the stage of liver disease, the response to therapy, and the potential availability of an IFN-free regimen.

DERMATOLOGIC COMPLICATIONS

Dry skin and pruritus are the most common IFN-related dermatologic side effects, seriously affecting patients' skin barrier, quality of life, and sleep. A break in the skin can become the port of entry for a bacterial infection if not treated with good skin hygiene.[23,24]

Table 6
Pegylated interferon dose modification for depression

Depression Severity	Dose Modification
Mild	No change
Moderate	Decrease dose 50%
Severe	Discontinue

Injection site reactions may occur, but rarely require cessation of therapy. These are typically characterized by local tenderness, erythema, and itching; skin necrosis and infection are rare, but must be addressed with topical steroid cream management.[25]

The cause of drug rash is multifactorial and can be related to IFN, RBV, or any concomitant medication. It is prudent to eliminate any unnecessary medications before HCV therapy and to recommend good skin hygiene to prevent local skin break-down. For patients who develop drug-related rash, use of topical antipruritics, anti-inflammatory agents, or systemic antihistamines can be beneficial. Telaprevir, when combined with IFN and RBV, is associated with rash in approximately 50% of patients; the development of severe rash may lead to drug discontinuation in approximately 5% of patients.[26]

An erythematous, eczematous rash in sun-exposed areas may be an RBV-associated photosensitivity; patients should avoid sun exposure and use sunscreen cream during RBV therapy.[27]

Patients with autoimmune diseases, such as psoriasis, are at risk for exacerbation of their dermatologic skin condiritos during IFN therapy; treatment interruption may be necessary, especially if systemic manifestations are present.[2,28]

Alopecia can occur in a subset of patients during the course of IFN therapy, and is probably another exacerbation of an autoimmune disease.[29] If the early virologic response is favorable patients should be encouraged to continue their treatment because hair loss is reversible after therapy is discontinued.

Some of the cutaneous manifestations of HCV infection, such as cryoglobulienemia, often get better as HCV RNA is suppressed.[30] There are reports that porphyria cutanea tarda can become exacerbated during RBV therapy initially, but can subsequently improve with sustained clearance of HCV infection.[31]

PULMONARY COMPLICATIONS

The pulmonary complications of HCV therapy are IFN-related and manifest as pneumonia and interstitial pneumonitis; pre-existing immune-related exacerbations can be prevented with a thorough screening before treatment. IFN therapy may also lead to the exacerbation of sarcoidosis and is contraindicated in this setting.[32]

If the patient presents with persistent dry cough without dyspnea on exertion that becomes gradually worse with no apparent chest radiograph findings, interstitial pneumonitis should be ruled out using a chest high-resolution CT scan imaging. If interstitial pneumonitis is diagnosed, IFN should be discontinued because symptoms are reversible after the withdrawal of IFN therapy.[33] The use of noninvasive imaging modalities, in combination with pulmonary function evaluation, can help the clinician decide whether or not to stop IFN therapy (see **Table 2**).

CARDIOVASCULAR COMPLICATIONS

The most common vascular events reported during CAH C therapy are related to the severity of anemia and underlying cardiovascular risk factors.[34,35] In patients with CAD, the authors recommend a prior stress test and optimization of cardiovascular status before therapy.

The HCV provider should have a lower threshold for dose reduction of RBV first and, if needed, IFN, to keep the hemoglobin level more than 12 g/dL in patients who are at risk for CAD (see **Table 3**).

A much rarer cardiac complication is cardiomyopathy, mainly reported in patients receiving higher doses of IFN for neoplastic disorders, which is reversible after cessation of therapy.[36]

GASTROINTESTINAL AES

Some of the most frequently reported gastrointestinal symptoms include nausea and boceprevir-associated dysgeusia. Neither of these symptoms plays a major factor in treatment interruption, but is vital to recognize to preserve the quality of life so patients may adhere to their therapy. Patients may minimize nausea when they take their RBV with food; however, antiemetics may be needed for a short period of time.

Epigastric pain may occur, possibly related to NSAID use for treatment or prophylaxis of flulike symptoms and can be managed by changing NSAIDs to acetaminophen, or by adding a proton-pump inhibitor if symptoms persist after NSAIDs are stopped. If the epigastric pain is very severe, amylase and lipase should be drawn to exclude drug-induced pancreatitis, a rare complication of IFN therapy. All cases of drug-induced pancreatitis occurred in the first few weeks of therapy and resolved with discontinuation of IFN-RBV.[37–39]

Patients presenting with a rectal bleed and abdominal pain should be worked-up for ischemic colitis, an unusual complication of IFN therapy. Ischemic colitis can be diagnosed by CT scan with contrast or colonoscopy. IFN should be discontinued in patients with this complication.[40]

Autoimmune disorders, such as inflammatory bowel disorders, may flare up or be uncovered during therapy. IFN is relatively contraindicated in such patients.[41] IFN is also contraindicated in patients with autoimmune hepatitis. Baseline screening (Antinuclear antibody [ANA] and Anti-smooth muscle antibody; if either is positive and autoimmune hepatitis is suspected, the following should be ordered: anti-liver-Kidney microsomal antibody type1, Anti-Mitochondrial antibody, p-anti-neutrophilic cytoplasmic antibody) for autoimmune hepatitis guides the use of IFN in treatment.

Mild abnormalities of aminotransferases during the treatment of chronic HCV with IFN and RBV are common, usually asymptomatic, and rarely lead to discontinuation of therapy. These liver enzyme elevations of aspartate transaminase and alanine transaminase are associated with greater pretreatment body weight, hepatic steatosis, and lower SVR rates.

Patients with poorly compensated liver disease are poor candidates for IFN, which may lead to decompensated liver disease and development of ascites, and liver-related death. IFN is contraindicated in those with decompensated cirrhosis with a Child-Pugh score greater than six.[42]

AUTOIMMUNE COMPLICATIONS
Thyroid

Thyroid abnormalities, frequently encountered during therapy, are considered part of the autoimmune side effects of IFN.[43] Thyroid autoantibodies are often detected in patients with chronic active hepatitis C even before therapy, especially in women, and they increase the risk for thyroid dysfunction during therapy. It is recommended to check thyroid-stimulating hormone at baseline, then every 3 months while on therapy and in the presence of symptoms of either hypothyroidism or hyperthyroidism.[28,44]

Patients who develop hypothyroidism should receive hormone replacement therapy. In contrast, patients developing hyperthyroidism should be evaluated by an endocrinologist for further management. Decisions about the continuation of IFN depend on a risk-benefit ratio calculated based on liver histology, response to therapy, availability of an IFN-free regimen, and the severity of the symptoms of hyperthyroidism.

New-onset diabetes mellitus with the presence of islet cell antibodies may rarely appear as a complication of IFN therapy.[45]

Other Autoimmune Disorders

There are several autoimmune disorders that may flare up or appear during IFN therapy, such as psoriasis, thyroiditis, autoimmune hepatitis, sarcoidosis, and inflammatory bowel disorders (**Table 7**). Hemolytic anemia, systemic lupus erythematosus, and idiopathic thrombocytopenic purpura have been reported and should be considered in the differential diagnosis in the appropriate clinical settings, when drug modifications do not improve laboratory markers.

For instance, a hemolytic anemia that does not improve with RBV dose reduction, or TCP that does not improve after IFN dose reduction, should trigger an autoimmune work-up. Most autoimmune conditions seem to abate after withdrawal of IFN, but it some cases treatment with steroids or other immunosuppressive therapy may be required.[46,47]

TERATOGENICITY

RBV-associated teratogenicity must be addressed in all males and females of child bearing capability. Pregnancy testing is indicated at baseline and subsequently at each visit.[10] Confirmation that a male patient's partner is not currently pregnant should be performed, and if a male patient's female partner is pregnant, he must wait until after delivery to begin therapy. Two forms of birth control, such as condoms with oral contraceptives, are recommended during therapy and up to 6 months after discontinuation of RBV.

MISCELLANEOUS
Drug-Drug Interactions

Notable drug interactions that should be cautioned with IFN are theophylline and methadone. With IFN, theophylline area under the curve was increased by 25%, because of inhibition of CYP1A2, and methadone level was mildly increased.[30]

With RBV an increased level of didanosine was described and as a result both drugs should not be coadministered because they increase mitochondrial toxicity. This combination is associated with increased mortality in Pegasys' registration trial for coinfected patients.[30,44]

Table 7	
Autoimmune exacerbations and their diagnosis	
Autoimmune Condition	**How to Diagnose?**
Psoriasis	Usually pre-existing Dermatologic evaluation
Inflammatory bowel disorders	Colonoscopy with biopsy
Thyroiditis	Anti-TPO Abs
Autoimmune hepatitis	Anti–smooth muscle Ab
Sarcoidosis	Pulmonary function tests, CT scan
Systemic lupus erythematosus	ANA, RF
Idiopathic thrombocytopenic purpura	Antiplatelet Abs

Abbreviations: Ab, Antibody; ANA, Antinuclear antibody; RF, Rheumatoid Factor; TPO, Anti-Thyroid Peroxidase.

Hypersensitivity Reactions

Hypersensitivity reactions (eg, urticaria, angioedema, bronchoconstriction, and anaphylaxis) have been rarely observed during IFN therapy. If a hypersensitivity reaction develops, discontinue treatment and institute appropriate medical therapy immediately for symptomatic relief. Transient rashes do not necessitate interruption of treatment.[42]

SUMMARY

The treatment of HCV with IFN and RBV should be undertaken by physicians with a broad clinical knowledge with close clinical follow-up of patients to avoid harm. If recognized early and treated appropriately most of the side effects of HCV therapy can be managed effectively by the provider.

Prescreening patients for potential clinical problems is vital to anticipating any AEs and involving specialists in a timely manner. Twice monthly visits in the beginning of therapy ensure that the HCV provider is able to address side effects as early as possible, while monitoring the efficacy of the regimen. Subsequent visits are guided by the patient's tolerability of the treatment and pre-existing comorbidities, although most patients should be seen every 4 weeks until the end of therapy if they are stable.

REFERENCES

1. Aspinall RJ, Pockros PJ. The management of side-effects during therapy for hepatitis C. Aliment Pharmacol Ther 2004;20(9):917–29.
2. Fried MW, Shiffman ML, Reddy KR, et al. Peginterferon alfa-2a plus ribavirin for chronic hepatitis C virus infection. N Engl J Med 2002;347(13):975–82.
3. Global Burden of Hepatitis C Working Group. Global burden of disease (GBD) for hepatitis C. J Clin Pharmacol 2004;44(1):20–9.
4. Hadziyannis SJ, Sette H Jr, Morgan TR, et al, PEGASYS International Study Group. Peginterferon-alpha2a and ribavirin combination therapy in chronic hepatitis C: a randomized study of treatment duration and ribavirin dose. Ann Intern Med 2004;140(5):346–55.
5. Russo MW, Fried MW. Side effects of therapy for chronic hepatitis C. Gastroenterology 2003;124(6):1711–9.
6. Torriani FJ, Rodriguez-Torres M, Rockstroh JK, et al, APRICOT Study Group. Peginterferon Alfa-2a plus ribavirin for chronic hepatitis C virus infection in HIV-infected patients. N Engl J Med 2004;351(5):438–50.
7. Fattovich G, Giustina G, Favarato S, et al. A survey of adverse events in 11,241 patients with chronic viral hepatitis treated with alfa interferon. J Hepatol 1996;24: 38–47.
8. McHutchison JG, Dusheiko G, Shiffman ML, et al. Eltrombopag for thrombocytopenia in patients with cirrhosis associated with hepatitis C. N Engl J Med 2007; 357:2227–36.
9. Dourakis SP, Deutsch M, Hadziyannis SJ. Immune thrombocytopenia and alpha-interferon therapy. J Hepatol 1996;25:972–5.
10. Kraus MR, Schafer A, Schottker K, et al. Therapy of interferon-induced depression in chronic hepatitis C with citalopram: a randomised, double-blind, placebo-controlled study. Gut 2008;57:531–6.
11. Ong JP, Younossi ZM. Managing the hematologic side effects of antiviral therapy for chronic hepatitis C: anemia, neutropenia, and thrombocytopenia. Cleve Clin J Med 2004;71(Suppl 3):S17–21.

12. Watanabe U, Hashimoto E, Hisamitsu T, et al. The risk factor for development of thyroid disease during interferon-alpha therapy for chronic hepatitis C. Am J Gastroenterol 1994;89:399–403.

13. Deutsch M, Dourakis S, Manesis EK, et al. Thyroid abnormalities in chronic viral hepatitis and their relationship to interferon alfa therapy. Hepatology 1997;26: 206–10.

14. Tran A, Quaranta JF, Benzaken S, et al. High prevalence of thyroid autoantibodies in a prospective series of patients with chronic hepatitis C before interferon therapy. Hepatology 1993;18:253–7.

15. Marazuela M, Garcia-Buey L, Gonzalez-Fernandez B, et al. Thyroid autoimmune disorders in patients with chronic hepatitis C before and during interferon-alpha therapy. Clin Endocrinol (Oxf) 1996;44:635–42.

16. Fabris P, Betterle C, Greggio NA, et al. Insulin-dependent diabetes mellitus during alphainterferon therapy for chronic viral hepatitis. J Hepatol 1998;28: 514–7.

17. Descamps V. Cutaneous side effects of alpha interferon. Presse Med 2005;34: 1668–72.

18. Lubbe J, Kerl K, Negro F, et al. Clinical and immunological features of hepatitis C treatment-associated dermatitis in 36 prospective cases. Br J Dermatol 2005; 153:1088–90.

19. Berk DR, Mallory SB, Keeffe EB, et al. Dermatologic disorders associated with chronic hepatitis C: effect of interferon therapy. Clin Gastroenterol Hepatol 2007;5:142–51.

20. Lang AM, Norland AM, Schuneman RL, et al. Localized interferon alfa-2b-induced alopecia. Arch Dermatol 1999;135:1126–8.

21. Kanazawa K, Yaoita H, Tsuda F, et al. Association of prurigo with hepatitis C virus infection. Arch Dermatol 1995;131:852–3.

22. Khella SL, Frost S, Hermann GA, et al. Hepatitis C infection, cryoglobulinemia, and vasculitic neuropathy. Treatment with interferon alfa: case report and literature review. Neurology 1995;45:407–11.

23. Stubgen JP. Interferon alpha and neuromuscular disorders. J Neuroimmunol 2009;207:3–17.

24. Weegink CJ, Chamuleau RA, Reesink HW, et al. Development of myasthenia gravis during treatment of chronic hepatitis C with interferon-alpha and ribavirin. J Gastroenterol 2001;36:723–4.

25. Karim A, Ahmed S, Khan A, et al. Interstitial pneumonitis in a patient treated with alpha-interferon and ribavirin for hepatitis C infection. Am J Med Sci 2001;322:233–5.

26. Jain K, Lam WC, Waheeb S, et al. Retinopathy in chronic hepatitis C patients during interferon treatment with ribavirin. Br J Ophthalmol 2001;85:1171–3.

27. Dereure O, Raison-Peyron N, Larrey D, et al. Diffuse inflammatory lesions in patients treated with interferon alfa and ribavirin for hepatitis C: a series of 20 patients. Br J Dermatol 2002;147:1142–6.

28. Manns MP, McHutchison JG, Gordon SC, et al. Peginterferon alfa-2b plus ribavirin compared with interferon alfa-2b plus ribavirin for initial treatment of chronic hepatitis C: a randomized trial. Lancet 2001;358:958–65.

29. Peg-Intron (peginterferon alfa-2b). [package insert]. Kelinworth (NJ): Schering Corporation; 2005. Available at: http://www.spfiles.com/pipeg-intron.pdf. Accessed June 15, 2008.

30. Pegasys (peginterferon alfa-2a). [package insert]. Nutley (NJ): Hoffmann-La Roche Inc.; 2002. Available at: http://pegasys.com/hcp/default.aspx. Accessed June 15, 2008.

31. Kartal ED, Colak H, Ozgunes I, et al. Exacerbation of psoriasis due to peginterferon alfa-2b plus ribavirin treatment of chronic active hepatitis C. Chemotherapy 2005;51:167–9.
32. Kartal ED, Alpat SN, Ozgunes I, et al. Reversible alopecia universalis secondary to PEG-interferon alfa-2b and ribavirin combination therapy in a patient with chronic hepatitis C virus infection. Eur J Gastroenterol Hepatol 2007;19:817–20.
33. Stryjek-Kaminska D, Ochsendorf F, Roder C, et al. Photoallergic skin reaction to ribavirin. Am J Gastroenterol 1999;94:1686–8.
34. Punnam SR, Pothula VR, Gourineni N, et al. Interferon-ribavirin-associated ischemic colitis. J Clin Gastroenterol 2008;42:323–5.
35. Tursi A. Rapid onset of ulcerative colitis after treatment with PEG-interferon plus ribavirin for chronic hepatitis C. Inflamm Bowel Dis 2007;13:1189–90.
36. Ozdogan O, Tahan V, Cincin A, et al. Acute pancreatitis associated with the use of peginterferon. Pancreas 2007;34:485–7.
37. Renou C, Germain S, Harafa A, et al. Interstitial pneumonia recurrence during chronic hepatitis C treatment. Am J Gastroenterol 2005;100:1625–6.
38. Kee KM, Lee CM, Wang JH, et al. Thyroid dysfunction in patients with chronic hepatitis C receiving a combined therapy of interferon and ribavirin: incidence, associated factors and prognosis. J Gastroenterol Hepatol 2006;21:319–26.
39. Yan KK, Dinihan I, Freiman J, et al. Sarcoidosis presenting with granulomatous uveitis induced by pegylated interferon and ribavirin therapy for hepatitis C. Intern Med J 2008;38(3):207–10.
40. Condat B, Asselah T, Zanditenas D, et al. Fatal cardiomyopathy associated with pegylated interferon/ribavirin in a patient with chronic hepatitis C. Eur J Gastroenterol Hepatol 2006;18:287–9.
41. Doyle MK, Berggren R, Magnus JH. Interferon-induced sarcoidosis. J Clin Rheumatol 2006;12:241–8.
42. Dieperink E, Ho SB, Tetrick L, et al. Suicidal ideation during interferon-alpha2b and ribavirin treatment of patients with chronic hepatitis C. Gen Hosp Psychiatry 2004;26:237–40.
43. Lodato F, Tame MR, Colecchia A, et al. Systemic lupus erythematosus following virological response to peginterferon alfa-2b in a transplanted patient with chronic hepatitis C recurrence. World J Gastroenterol 2006;12:4253–5.
44. Mauss S, Valenti W, DePamphilis J, et al. Risk factors for heptatic decompensation in patients with HIV/HCV coinfection and liver cirrhosis during interferon-based therapy. AIDS 2004;18:F21–5.
45. McHutchinson JG, Lawitz EJ, Shiffman ML, et al. Peginterferon alfa-2b or alfa-2a with ribavirin for treatment of hepatitis C infection. N Engl J Med 2009;361:580–93.
46. Reddy KR, Shiffman ML, Morgan TR, et al. Impact of ribavirin dose reductions in hepatitis C virus genotype 1 patients completing peginterferon alfa-2a/ribavirin treatment. Clin Gastroenterol Hepatol 2007;5:124–9.
47. Sulkowski MS, Shiffman ML, Afdhal NH, et al. Hepatitis C virus treatment-related anemia is associated with higher sustained virologic response rate. Gastroenterology 2010;139:1602–11.

Treatment of Hepatitis C in Patients Infected with Human Immunodeficiency Virus in the Direct-Acting Antiviral Era

Vincent Soriano, MD, PhD*, Pablo Labarga, MD, PhD,
Eugenia Vispo, MD, José Vicente Fernández-Montero, MD, PhD,
Pablo Barreiro, MD, PhD

KEYWORDS

- Hepatitis C • Direct-acting antivirals • HIV • Coinfection • Drug resistance
- Drug interactions • Telaprevir • Boceprevir

KEY POINTS

- Chronic hepatitis C virus (HCV) infection affects globally 25% of HIV-infected individuals worldwide. The prevalence is higher among intravenous drug users than subjects infected sexually.
- Progression of liver disease is faster in HIV-HCV coinfected versus HCV-monoinfected individuals. Thus, treatment of hepatitis C must be encouraged in coinfected patients.
- New oral direct-acting antivirals (DAA) are currently being added to peginterferon/ribavirin, providing rates of HCV cure above 70%.
- DAA combinations are eagerly awaited by HIV-HCV coinfected patients. They will be given soon in combinations without interferon and for shorter treatment periods (12-24 weeks).
- Drug-drug interactions and side effects challenge the use of DAA in HIV-HCV coinfected patients.

INTRODUCTION

Liver disease is currently one of the leading causes of hospitalization and death in people infected with human immunodeficiency virus (HIV) in the western world.[1,2] AIDS-related opportunistic infections and cancers have steadily declined and are currently diagnosed, mainly in individuals who are unaware of their HIV status and/ or among recent immigrants from highly HIV-endemic developing regions where anti-retroviral therapy is not easily available. For most patients infected with HIV in

Department of Infectious Diseases, Hospital Carlos III, Madrid, Spain
* Corresponding author. Department of Infectious Diseases, Hospital Carlos III, Calle Sinesio Delgado 10, Madrid 28029, Spain.
E-mail address: vsoriano@dragonet.es

Infect Dis Clin N Am 26 (2012) 931–948
http://dx.doi.org/10.1016/j.idc.2012.08.004
0891-5520/12/$ – see front matter © 2012 Elsevier Inc. All rights reserved.

developed countries who regular attend HIV outpatient clinics, hepatic complications result mainly from chronic viral hepatitis, drug-related hepatotoxicity (antiretrovirals and other medications), alcohol abuse, or fatty liver disease (**Box 1**).[3,4]

Chronic hepatitis C is by far the most frequent cause of liver complications in patients infected with HIV parenterally (ie, intravenous drug users or recipients of contaminated blood or blood products). More than two-thirds of intravenous drug users with HIV infection in Europe and North America have chronic hepatitis C.[5,6] **Box 2** summarizes the main characteristics of hepatitis C virus (HCV) infection. In the absence of successful HCV therapy, one-third may progress to cirrhosis within 25 years of infection,[5] a rate significantly faster than in HCV-monoinfected individuals. The accelerated progression of liver disease in the HIV setting may be ameliorated with the use of highly active antiretroviral therapy (HAART),[7] which has led to earlier initiation of antiretroviral treatment in all individuals coinfected with HIV and HCV.[6,8] Even so, accumulated toxicity from antiretroviral drugs and HIV itself or comorbidities (ie, metabolic abnormalities) explain why progression of HCV-related liver disease still remains accelerated in most coinfected patients on HAART.[9]

TREAT HCV OR HIV FIRST?

Underlying chronic hepatitis C enhances the risk of increases in liver enzymes in patients using HAART,[10,11] and the tolerance of antiretroviral therapy improves after clearance of HCV with successful therapy.[12] Thus, in the absence of contraindications, treatment of chronic hepatitis C should be provided as early as possible to coinfected persons. Ideally, it might be considered before beginning antiretroviral therapy in patients with CD4 counts >500 cells/μL and relatively low plasma HIV-RNA (ie, <50,000 copies/mL). If plasma HIV-RNA is greater, concerns have been raised about a detrimental effect of uncontrolled HIV replication on the efficacy of hepatitis C therapy.[13]

TREATMENT OF COINFECTED PATIENTS

In places where interferon α (IFNα)-based HCV therapy has been widely used in patients coinfected with HIV and HCV, those who are not cured often show a difficult-to-treat phenotype, characterized by high HCV-RNA levels, infection by HCV genotypes 1 or 4,[14] unfavorable IL28B alleles, and/or advanced liver fibrosis. **Fig. 1** records the current profile of 414 individuals infected with HIV with active HCV replication in 2011 in a referral clinic in Spain.[15] Therapeutic options for this population are limited and many coinfected patients with advanced liver fibrosis have already died and/or entered liver transplant lists, although only a few have received a transplant.[16] Moreover, liver transplantation is not the ultimate solution for patients coinfected with HIV and HCV, given that HCV reinfection of the allograft is almost

---

Box 1
Main causes of liver damage in patients infected with HIV

- Viral hepatitis (B, C, D, E)
- Metabolic abnormalities, nonalcoholic steatohepatitis
- Alcohol abuse
- Drug-related hepatotoxicity
- Liver involvement in other conditions, such as infections (ie, tuberculosis) or cancers (ie, lymphoma)

Box 2
Hepatitis C worldwide

- 2% of the world population (175 million people)
- 1.5% in the West (~40% undiagnosed)
- Routes of infection: sporadic >50%
- Risk factors: transfusions before 1990; intravenous drug use
- 30% of chronic carriers will develop cirrhosis
- HCV is the primary reason for liver transplantation
- HCV is the major cause of liver cancer in the West
- No vaccine
- Only curable (eradicable) chronic viral infection

---

universal and progression to cirrhosis is further accelerated in HIV/HCV-coinfected transplanted patients, with survival rates less than 50% at 5 years after transplantation.[17] Novel anti-HCV therapies are urgently needed in this population.

LESSONS FROM USING DIRECT-ACTING ANTIVIRALS IN HCV MONOINFECTION

The treatment of HCV infection is evolving rapidly after the arrival of the first HCV protease inhibitors. Telaprevir and boceprevir were approved by US and European agencies in 2011 for the treatment of chronic hepatitis C genotype 1 infection in combination with pegylated interferon alpha (pegIFNα) and ribavirin (RBV).

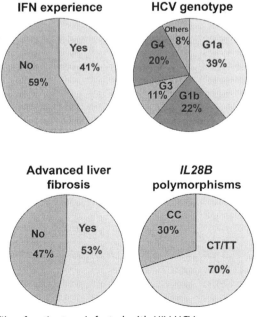

Fig. 1. Current profile of patients coinfected with HIV-HCV.

For treatment-naive patients and prior relapsers, telaprevir is given orally 750 mg (2 pills)/8 hours for the first 12 weeks of therapy, continuing with pegIFNα/RBV for an additional 12 weeks (total duration of therapy 24 weeks) among those who achieve undetectable HCV-RNA at week 4 of therapy (RVR, rapid virologic response). For those who do not achieve RVR, pegIFNα/RBV is continued for an additional 36 weeks (total duration of therapy 48 weeks). The sustained virological response rate observed in treatment-naive HCV-monoinfected patients ranged from 44% in pegIFNα/RBV controls to 75% in telaprevir triple therapy arms.[18] However, telaprevir is associated with a higher treatment discontinuation rate due to adverse effects, of which rash is the most common and can be severe in up to nearly 5% of patients. Other frequent adverse events are gastrointestinal side effects (nausea, vomiting, diarrhea), pruritus, and anemia.[19,20] Given the challenge represented by the need for dosing the drug 3 times daily, the results of a recent study on HCV-monoinfected patients supporting twice daily dosing of telaprevir[21] are especially welcome, although there are no similar data for the coinfected population.

Boceprevir is another linear serine HCV protease inhibitor approved for use in combination with pegIFNα/RBV in patients infected with HCV genotype 1. In phase III trials, sustained virological response rates of 67% to 68% were obtained in boceprevir arms compared with 40% in pegIFN/RBV controls in IFNα-naive white patients.[22] These figures were 69% to 75% versus 29% in prior relapsers and 40% to 52% versus 7% in prior partial responders; null responders were excluded.[23] In all boceprevir treatment arms, however, there was a significantly increased risk of anemia compared with pegIFNα/RBV, and erythropoetin was used by 40% of patients. No severe rash has been reported with boceprevir. Similar to telaprevir, boceprevir patients with viral breakthrough or relapse select for viruses with drug-resistant mutations. As with telaprevir, relapses are seen in less than 10% of patients treated with boceprevir, whereas it is around 25% in patients treated only with pegIFNα/RBV.

Other molecules with potent antiviral activity, an improved safety profile, and more convenient dosing are being tested in clinical trials and it is hoped they will come to market soon (**Table 1**). Most direct-acting antivirals (DAAs) target specific HCV enzymes, such as the polymerase, protease, or the NS5A protein. To date, only a few phase I and II studies have been performed with these newer agents in patients infected with HIV and further investigations must be encouraged.

Table 1
DAAs in more advanced stages of clinical development

| Protease Inhibitors | Polymerase Inhibitors | | NS5A Inhibitors |
	Nucleos(t)ide Analogues	Non-nucleoside Analogues	
Telaprevir	Mericitabine	Tegobuvir	Daclatasvir
Boceprevir	GS-7977	Filibuvir	GS-5885
Simeprevir	IDX-184	BI-7127	IDX-179
Danoprevir	INX-189	BI-1325	ABT-267
Vaniprevir		Setrobuvir	
BI-1335		VX-222	
MK-5172		VCH-759	
GS-9256		ABT-072	
ABT-450		GS-9669	
ACH-1625			

PREDICTORS OF RESPONSE TO DAA THERAPY

Besides the classic predictors of response to hepatitis C therapy (ie, HCV genotype, baseline serum HCV-RNA, and liver fibrosis stage), emergent data support that other new variables may influence treatment response using DAAs (**Table 2**). For example, it is remarkable that HCV subtype 1a viruses respond less well to most of the new agents compared with HCV subtype 1b. As an illustrative example, **Fig. 2** records the viral response to triple therapy including simeprevir (TMC-435), an HCV protease inhibitor in the latest stages of clinical development. Patients harboring subtype 1a responded less well than those with subtype 1b.[24] Furthermore, it is intriguing why unfavorable IL28B alleles still exert a deleterious effect on response to IFN-free oral combinations.[25]

Baseline polymorphisms at positions associated with resistance to some DAAs may be relevant and influence antiviral responses. An example is a change at protease codon 80, which may compromise the response to low doses of simeprevir (**Fig. 3**).[24] As shown in **Table 3**, Q80K is present in around 40% of HCV-1a strains. If this variable is proved to influence the response to other antivirals, baseline drug resistance testing may be beneficial as seen with HIV therapy; however, baseline HCV drug resistance testing is currently not recommended.

EVALUATION OF DAAS IN THE HIV SETTING

Drug interactions with HIV antiretroviral medications,[26,27] increased and overlapping toxicities, and rapid selection of drug-resistant HCV mutants are among the most challenging issues with the use of DAAs in patients coinfected with HIV and HCV.[28] This is further complicated because other recently identified prognostic factors also play a role in the outcome of HCV treatment in patients coinfected with HIV and HCV. As seen in HCV monoinfection, polymorphisms at the host IL28B gene strongly predict treatment success in coinfected patients.[29,30] Insulin resistance is another variable that compromises treatment response, and it is common in coinfected patients.[31,32] CD4 counts and HIV replication are unique to the coinfected patient and need to be considered in any trial design of HCV therapy in this population.

TELAPREVIR IN COINFECTED PATIENTS

The first data on the use of telaprevir in patients coinfected with HIV and HCV were recently released.[33] Vertex study 110 was a phase II study that examined the safety and efficacy of telaprevir in combination with pegIFNα/RBV compared with standard therapy alone in 60 patients coinfected with HIV and HCV, a quarter of whom were not taking antiretroviral therapy. Given the induction of telaprevir metabolism by efavirenz,

| Table 2 | |
| Predictors of HCV treatment response | |
Old	**New**
HCV genotype	IL28B alleles
Viral load	Baseline drug resistance HCV polymorphisms
Liver fibrosis	HCV-1 subtypes
Rapid virological response	
Drug adherence	
Anemia	

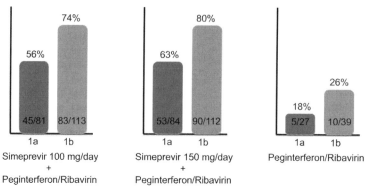

Fig. 2. Sustained virological response to triple therapy including simeprevir, according to HCV subtype 1a or 1b.

higher telaprevir dosing (1125 mg every 8 hours) was used in patients receiving efavirenz. Other antiretrovirals allowed in the trial were tenofovir, emtricitabine, lamivudine, and ritonavir-boosted atazanavir, for all of which information on drug interactions is available. At week 12 after the discontinuation of HCV therapy, viral suppression rates were significantly higher among patients on triple therapy compared with dual therapy (74% vs 45%) (**Fig. 4**). Three individuals discontinued triple therapy prematurely because of side effects. Rash developed in one-third of patients treated with telaprevir, although none was severe. Hyperbilirubinemia was exacerbated in patients on atazanavir/r because of increased atazanavir exposure by telaprevir.

BOCEPREVIR IN COINFECTED PATIENTS

The phase II trial that tested boceprevir triple therapy in HIV/HCV coinfection included 98 patients.[34] As in the telaprevir trial, all were interferon naive and infected by HCV genotype 1 strains. Patients were randomly assigned 2:1 to triple therapy versus pegIFN/RBV. **Fig. 5** shows the virological response in the 2 groups at different time points. It is intriguing that only a minority of patients achieved a rapid virologic response and the peak maximal response in the triple arm occurred at week 24,

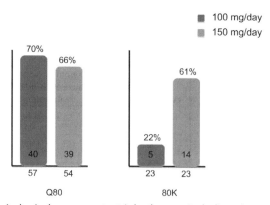

Fig. 3. Sustained virological response to triple therapy including simeprevir, based on the presence of Q80K at the HCV protease.

Table 3
Natural polymorphisms influencing DAA susceptibility

Drug Family	Key Mutations Associated with DAA Resistance*	1a	1b	2	3	4	DAA Affected by Specific Polymorphisms
NS3 protease inhibitors (no. of NS3 sequences: 1612†)	T54A/S	1.4% S	0	0	0	5.5% S	Telaprevir, boceprevir
	V55A	1.2% A	0	0	0	0	Boceprevir
	Q80K	39.7% K	0	0	0	0	Simeprevir
	D168A/H/T/V/Q	0	0	0	99.2% Q	0	Simeprevir
NS5B non- nucleoside analogues (no. of NS5B sequences: 1025†)	C316Y/N	0	36% N	0	0	0	ABT-333 (NNI-4) ABT-072 (NNI-4)
	M414T/L	0	0	0	0	34.2% L	Setrobuvir (NNI-3)
	L419M/V	0	0	2.7% V	0	0	VCH-759 (NNI-2)
	M423T/I/V	1.8 I	0	0	0	0	Filibuvir (NNI-2) VCH-759 (NNI-2) VHC-916 (NNI-2)
	I482L/V/T	0	0	100% L	100% L	100% L	VCH-759 (NNI-2)
	V494I/A	0	0	100% A	5.2% A	0	VCH-759 (NNI-2)
	V499A**	96.2% A	10.5% A	91% A	100% A	100% A	Tegobuvir (NNI-1) BI-7127 (NNI-1)
NS5a inhibitors (no. of NS5a sequences: 3153†)	Q30H/R	0	0	0	0	51.3% R	Daclatasvir
	L31M/V/F	0	0	83.5% M	0	92% M	Daclatasvir
	Y93C/H/N	0	2% H	0	0	5.4% H	Daclatasvir

* Only changes with a prevalence >1% are recorded.
** V499A confers low-level resistance to NNI-1.
† NS3 protease, NS5B polymerase and NS5A sequences were obtained from Los Alamos database.
No mutations associated with resistance to NS5B nucleos(t)ide analogues are found as natural polymorphisms.

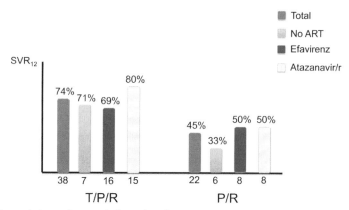

Fig. 4. Telaprevir in patients coinfected with HIV/HCV.

perhaps indirectly reflecting a limited activity of boceprevir in comparison with other HCV protease inhibitors (**Fig. 6**). Overall, the added benefit of triple therapy over standard of care ranged from 29% to 35%.

LIMITATIONS OF TRIPLE HCV THERAPY IN COINFECTED PATIENTS

The dosing schedule of first-generation HCV protease inhibitors lacks convenience, as both drugs must be given every 8 hours with food. There is also a significant pill burden as telaprevir has to be given as 2 pills (3 pills with efavirenz) and boceprevir as 4 pills for each dose. In HIV patients, this complex dosing must be integrated into the antiretroviral therapy requirement; for example, efavirenz should be taken on an empty stomach. Further, polypharmacy may be associated with poor drug adherence and this will be a major challenge in the treatment of chronic hepatitis C in individuals coinfected with HIV, as most patients are often taking other medications in addition to antiretroviral medications. Poor treatment adherence may lead to selection of drug resistance in HCV. Although the use of pegIFNα as part of hepatitis C therapy may suppress HIV replication ($\sim$1 log on average), poor drug compliance may increase the risk of failure to HCV protease inhibitors. Overlapping toxicities between HCV and HIV drugs (ie, rash, anemia) may have a further negative effect on the efficacy of HCV protease inhibitors in this population. Unexpected drug interactions between antivirals for HCV and HIV may result in reduced drug exposure and a tendency to

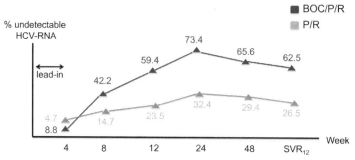

Fig. 5. Boceprevir in patients coinfected with HIV/HCV.

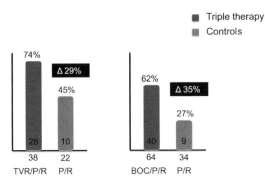

Fig. 6. SVR_{12} with boceprevir and telaprevir in patients coinfected with HIV/HCV.

virological failure. This is the case for most HIV protease inhibitors and non-nucleoside reverse transcriptase inhibitors, particularly boceprevir.

NO CROSS-ACTIVITY OR CROSS-RESISTANCE BETWEEN HIV AND HCV DRUGS

Because HIV and HCV share some biological similarities,[35] concern has been raised that HIV drugs might induce changes in the HCV polymerase and/or protease,[36] or vice versa. However, in a study of 28 patients coinfected with HIV and HCV in whom the HCV NS5B gene was sequenced before and during antiretroviral drug use, there was no evidence of selection of drug resistance mutations in the HCV polymerase.[37] It should be highlighted that the HCV polymerase is an RNA-dependent RNA polymerase distinct from the HIV reverse transcriptase, which is an RNA-dependent DNA polymerase, and that no cross-activity has been observed in vitro. Similarly, HCV protease is a serine protease, whereas HIV protease is a structurally different aspartate protease.[38] Thus, exposure to their respective antivirals does not select for resistance changes in the other virus.

DRUG INTERACTIONS BETWEEN DAA AND HIV MEDICATIONS

Most patients infected with HIV and chronic hepatitis C are receiving antiretroviral therapy. Moreover, as HIV patients become older, they often receive other medications for comorbidities, such as hypertension, dyslipidemia, diabetes, mood disorders, and so forth. Thus, the potential for drug interactions between DAA and concomitant medications must be checked before prescribing hepatitis C therapy. Whereas drug overexposure may increase toxicities, suboptimal exposure may cause treatment failure.[26,27]

Interactions Between pegIFNα/RBV and Antiretrovirals

Interactions between pegIFNα/RBV and ARVs are relatively limited, with concerns about RBV and zidovudine, didanosine, stavudine, or abacavir.[39–44] Hyperbilirubinemia may be more pronounced in patients taking RBV and atazanavir together.[45] For up-to-date information on HCV drug interactions, the reader can access the Web sites at http://www.hep-druginteractions.org and/or http://medicine.iupui.edu/clinpharm/ddis/.

Interactions Between HCV Protease Inhibitors and Antiretrovirals

Although data are still limited for many DAAs, a few have been well characterized and recommendations have been released.

Telaprevir

Telaprevir is a substrate and inhibitor of CYP3A4 and the transporter P-gp. Based on prior knowledge, it was assumed that telaprevir exposure would increase when coadministered with ritonavir-boosted HIV protease inhibitors.[26,27] Contrary to expectations, there is a reduction in telaprevir exposure, slight with atazanavir/r but significant with darunavir/r or fosamprenavir/r, and pronounced with lopinavir/r. The mechanism involved in the decreased exposure has yet to be determined (**Table 4**).

Efavirenz also reduces telaprevir exposure significantly, and an increased dose of telaprevir (1125 mg/8 hours) should be given, increasing the overall cost.[46] The use of tenofovir does not modify telaprevir exposure; however, telaprevir significantly increases tenofovir exposure and close monitoring of kidney function is warranted when both drugs are used concomitantly.[47] The effect of telaprevir on HIV protease inhibitors is variable, with reduced exposure for darunavir/r and fosamprenavir/r, no change for lopinavir/r, and increase for atazanavir/r trough concentrations.

Interactions between telaprevir and other frequent medications taken by individuals infected with HIV are recorded in **Table 5**. Telaprevir causes a decrease in the CYP2C9-metabolized antidepressant escitalopram.[48] The interactions of telaprevir with methadone[49] do not seem to be clinically relevant, because despite a decrease in the total R-methadone concentration, the unbound drug remains unaltered.

Boceprevir

Boceprevir is principally metabolized by the enzyme aldo-keto reductase with a minor contribution from CYP3A4; however, it inhibits CYP3A4.[50] Interaction studies on boceprevir were conducted in HIV-negative subjects using medications likely to be coadministered in patients with chronic hepatitis C.[51] The information recorded in **Table 4** suggests that CYP3A4 and P-gp do not contribute substantially to boceprevir metabolism and/or elimination.

There is no significant increase in boceprevir exposure when given with multiple doses of low-dose ritonavir (indeed there is a small decrease possibly due to induction). No dosage adjustment for boceprevir is needed when coadministered with tenofovir. The clinical implications of a reduced boceprevir trough concentration when coadministered with efavirenz are as yet unclear, but the current recommendation is to avoid this combination. To date, no information is available about interactions between boceprevir and raltegravir or methadone, although it is expected that they will not be clinically relevant.

Table 4
Interactions between DAAs and antiretrovirals

	Telaprevir Comedication		Boceprevir Comedication	
TDF	≈	↑30%	↑8%	↑8%
EFV	↓26% (tid)	↓7% (tid)	↓19%	↑20%
ATV/r	↓20%	↑17%	—	—
DRV/r	↓35%	↓40%	—	—
FPV/r	↓32%	↓47%	—	—
LPV/r	↓54%	↑6%	—	—
RTV (low dose)	↓24%	—	↓19%	—

Abbreviation: tid, 3 times a day.

Table 5
Interactions between DAAs and common medications

	Telaprevir Comedication		Boceprevir Comedication	
R-Methadone	≈	↓29%	—	—
Midazolam	—	9-fold	—	↑5-fold
Escitalopram	≈	↓35%	—	—
Esomeprazole	≈	—	—	—
Contraceptives (estrogen/ progestogen)	≈	↓28%/↓11%	—	↓24%/↑99%
Atorvastatin	—	↑8-fold	—	—
Ketoconazole	↑62%	↑46%	↑2.3-fold	—

Currently, boceprevir is only recommended for use with tenofovir, emtricitabine, and raltegravir. Recent information, however, suggests that etravirine, rilpivirine, and maraviroc can be safely coadministered with first-generation HCV protease inhibitors.

The aldo-keto reductase inhibitor diflusinal causes a small increase in boceprevir trough concentration. The increase in midazolam supports boceprevir as a strong reversible inhibitor of CYP3A4. Boceprevir significantly affects the exposure of the oral contraceptive drospirenone (increased) and ethinyloestradiol (decreased), and accordingly the use of these drugs along with boceprevir is contraindicated. The significance of the increase with progestogen is unclear (see **Table 5**).

Interactions Between HCV Polymerase Inhibitors and Antiretrovirals

The potential for pharmacokinetic interactions between HCV polymerase inhibitors and antiretrovirals is scarce. However, pharmacodynamic interactions may be more problematic, especially as a result of inhibitory competitive phenomena for drugs sharing their phosphorylation pathway. This has been demonstrated for mericitabine and other HIV cytidine analogues, such as lamivudine or emtricitabine.[27,28] Given that affinity binding for cellular kinases is higher for HIV drugs, mericitabine should not be prescribed along with lamivudine and/or emtricitabine.

HCV DRUG RESISTANCE IN THE HIV SETTING

One of the major challenges using DAAs is the risk of selective drug resistance, a concern that did not exist for pegIFNα or RBV. No doubt the knowledge about drug resistance in HIV is helpful for understanding resistance in HCV. However, biological differences between these viruses may account for distinct clinical implications.[35] At least 4 aspects have raised particular attention. First, the speed of selection of drug resistance in HCV is faster than in HIV, consistent with the low barrier to resistance of many HCV drugs (with the notable exception of nucleos(t)ide analogues inhibiting the active site of HCV polymerase).[52,53] The consequences are that there is no room for monotherapy (real or virtual) and that early viral kinetics (days to a few weeks) predict the likelihood of HCV treatment success.[54]

Second, as in HIV, broad cross-resistance between HCV drugs belonging to the same family exists,[55] with the exception of the non-nucleoside polymerase inhibitors.[56] The major positions associated with drug resistance are illustrated in **Fig. 7**. Given the high HCV variability, resistance patterns vary by the specific medication and HCV subtypes. For instance, after exposure to boceprevir and telaprevir, the most frequent resistance mutations are selected at codons 36 and 155 for HCV-1a and codons 54, 156, and 170 for HCV-1b.[57]

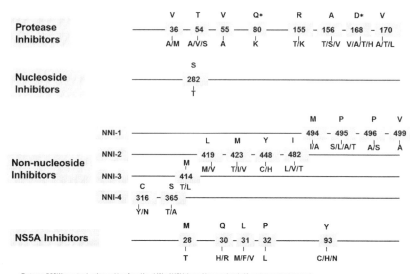

Fig. 7. Main drug resistance mutations to DAAs.

Third, transmission of drug-resistant viruses from patients infected with HCV may be less relevant than for patients with HIV, depending on whether patients with chronic hepatitis C exposed to DAAs who have failed therapy and have selective drug resistance remain engaged in high-risk behaviors, potentially becoming the source of new incident HCV cases. Sexual transmission of HCV is rare and many of the drug-resistant HCV strains revert back to wild-type within a few months after drug discontinuation.

In contrast, with HIV, natural polymorphisms across distinct HCV genotypes/ subtypes may be a huge challenge, driving differences in susceptibility to distinct DAAs and a barrier to resistance, and for this reason baseline resistance testing is justified. For instance, HCV protease codon Q80K polymorphism occurs in up to 40% of HCV subtype 1a, and this change has already been shown to compromise the response to simeprevir in a dose-dependent manner.[24]

Although concern has been raised about a potential harmful effect of HIV-associated immunodeficiency on the risk of selective drug resistance in HCV, as a result of increased variability caused by loss of immune control or interference with the concomitant use of antiretroviral agents, recent data do not support these concerns. As previously highlighted, viral enzyme targets for antivirals are different in HIV and HCV, and significant structural differences between these molecules preclude that treatment with their respective inhibitors may select drug resistance changes in the other virus.[37] On the other hand, viral diversity for HCV in the presence of immunosuppression does not seem to be associated with an increased rate of HCV resistance-associated mutations.[58,59]

SPECIAL HIV/HCV PATIENT POPULATIONS

There are groups of individuals coinfected with HIV and HCV with particular medical needs (Table 6). The highest need is for prior nonresponders to pegIFNα/RBV, patients intolerant to pegIFNα +/− RBV, individuals with advanced liver disease with thrombocytopenia and patients undergoing liver transplantation.

Table 6
Main challenges for DAAs in special HIV/HCV populations

Population	Caveat
Liver transplantation	Drug-drug interactions; rejection
Advanced liver disease (cirrhosis)	Impaired DAA metabolism; enhanced toxicity
Prior IFNα null responders	Lower response; increased risk for selecting HCV drug resistance
IFNα and/or RBV intolerant	Wait for IFN and/or RBV sparing combinations
Non-1 HCV genotypes	Poor or null activity for first-generation HCV protease inhibitors
Hemodialysis	No data
Children	Dose adjustments
Acute hepatitis C	No data; added value?
Inherited hematological disorders: thalassemia, hemophilia	Enhanced toxicities: anemia, bleeding
Socially dysfunctional groups (ie, homeless, illegal immigrants)	Difficult to reach and keep on satisfactory drug adherence
Intravenous drug users	Concerns about drug adherence and transmission of drug-resistant HCV mutants

Prior Interferon-α Nonresponders

In patients coinfected with HIV and HCV who failed a previous course of suboptimal hepatitis C therapy, retreatment with adequate doses and duration of pegIFNα/RBV should be considered in the presence of advanced liver fibrosis. But even with improved drug dosing, longer duration of treatment, and optimal adverse event management, the overall response rates in patients with HCV genotype 1 did not move up 20% in the best scenario. Successful treatment becomes even less likely if patients were previous null responders (<1 log drop in HCV-RNA on pegIFNα/RBV therapy). Most of these individuals harbor unfavorable IL28B alleles, and new therapeutic options are clearly needed for them. In the mean time, the use of a lead-in phase of pegIFNα/RBV may help to identify the subset of patients who will not benefit from triple therapy. This approach, originally developed in an attempt to reduce selective drug resistance to DAA, may now prove to be helpful to test pegIFNα susceptibility and tolerance (**Box 3**).

Advanced Liver Disease with Thrombocytopenia

Low platelet count in patients infected with HIV and HCV may be related to HIV or HCV. Thrombocytopenia associated with HIV infection generally improves after

Box 3
Usefulness of lead-in

- Original:
  - Reduce selection of drug resistance
- Current:
  - Test interferon susceptibility
  - Test IFN/RBV tolerance

suppression of viral replication with antiretroviral therapy. Low platelet count caused by HCV-related cirrhosis with portal hypertension and hypersplenism is more challenging, because pegIFNα therapy may enhance thrombocytopenia and increase the risk of bleeding. Clearly, other therapeutic options are eagerly awaited for this particularly difficult-to-treat population.

Liver Transplantation

The outcome of liver transplantation in patients infected with HIV is poorer than in individuals without HIV infection,[17] with 5-year survival rates of 48% versus 75%, respectively.[60] The main reason for this unfavorable prognosis is the accelerated course of the almost universal HCV reinfection of the allograft. The sustained virological response to pegIFNα/RBV is as low as 22% in liver transplant recipients coinfected with HIV and HCV. Clearly, better HCV treatment options are needed for this population; the major challenge is drug interactions between HIV and HCV drugs in the presence of immunosuppressants. Large increases in cyclosporine, and specially with tacrolimus exposure, were seen when coadministered with telaprevir.[61]

FUTURE PROSPECTS FOR DAAS IN HIV/HCV COINFECTION
Need for Interferon-Free Oral Combination Regimens

Contraindications for using either pegIFNα and/or RBV are common in individuals coinfected with HIV and HCV, and have discouraged the treatment of many patients until now. As DAAs will initially be provided along with pegIFNα/RBV, the benefit of triple therapy will still exclude certain populations, such as patients with serious neuropsychiatric conditions, decompensated cirrhosis, severe anemia, alcohol abuse, and renal disease. Unfortunately, all these situations are more frequently seen in coinfected than in HCV-monoinfected patients. Therefore, combination DAA regimens, sparing IFNα and/or RBV, are eagerly awaited for the treatment of chronic hepatitis C in the HIV population.

Personalized HCV Therapy in Coinfection

Given that the antiviral activity of DAA agents may differ according to HCV genotypes/subtypes (**Table 7**) and that the benefit of pegIFNα seems to be largely influenced by IL28B genotypes, it is reasonable to envisage that personalized regimens will progressively be advised.[62]

Table 7
Main differential features of new DAAs against HCV

	NS3 Protease Inhibitors	NS5B Polymerase Nucleos(t)ide Analogues	NS5B Polymerase Non-nucleoside Analogues	NS5A Inhibitors
Mechanism of inhibition	Inhibitory competition	Inhibitory competition	Allosteric	?
Genotype activity	G1 (G1b>G1a)	Across all	G1 (G1b>1a)	Across all (G1a<G1b)
Resistance barrier	Low	High	Low	Low
Cross-resistance	High	Low	Split out in 4–5 families	high
Drug interactions	PK	Pharmacodynamic	PK	PK

Box 4
Implications of widespread use of DAAs

- Significant increments in cost and demands for the health system, including well-trained personnel
- Shift in HCV genotypes within the infected population, being other genotypes replacing genotype 1
- Changes in HCV-infected populations, with accumulation in poor regions and/or marginalized communities within rich countries
- A growing number of patients with drug-resistant mutant viruses and potential for transmission

---

Implications of Widespread Use of DAAs in Coinfected Patients

After the approval of the first DAAs, widespread use of these agents should be expected. Their use will occasionally be off-label or under unsatisfactory medical conditions, which may result in undesirable toxicities, drug interactions, or selective drug resistance. On the other hand, the appropriate and judicious use of DAAs may provide a cure for a large number of patients. As a consequence, a growing proportion of the remaining infected patients will harbor non-1 HCV genotypes or drug-resistant HCV variants (**Box 4**).

Over time, the largest reservoir of patients with HCV will be concentrated in resource-poor nations where access to hepatitis C therapy has been elusive and HIV treatment remains the primary health issue for the coinfected population. In rich countries, HCV will rapidly become a disease of those with difficult access to the health system, a condition of marginalized individuals, such as the homeless, active intravenous drug users, alcoholics, illegal immigrants, and so forth.[62]

REFERENCES

1. Weber R, Sabin C, Friis-Møller N, et al. Liver-related deaths in persons infected with the HIV: the D: A:D study. Arch Intern Med 2006;166:1632–41.
2. Ruppik M, Ledergerber B, Rickenbach M, et al. Changing patterns of causes of death: SCCS, 2005 to 2009. Presented at CROI, Boston (MA), February 27–March 2, 2011 [abstract 789].
3. Merwat S, Vierling J. HIV infection and the liver: the importance of HCV-HIV coinfection and drug-induced liver injury. Clin Liver Dis 2011;15:131–52.
4. Peters M, Soriano V. HIV and the liver. In: Dooley J, Lok A, Burroughs A, et al, editors. Sherlock's diseases of the liver and biliary system. 12th edition. Oxford (United Kingdom): Blackwell Publishing Ltd; 2011. p. 438–51.
5. Soriano V, Puoti M, Sulkowski M, et al. Care of patients coinfected with HIV and hepatitis C virus: 2007 updated recommendations from the HCV-HIV International Panel. AIDS 2007;21:1073–89.
6. European AIDS Clinical Society (EACS) guidelines, October 2011. Available at: www.europeanaidsclinicalsociety.org. Accessed August 28, 2012.
7. Qurishi N, Kreuzberg C, Luchters G, et al. Effect of antiretroviral therapy on liver-related mortality in patients with HIV and hepatitis C virus coinfection. Lancet 2003;362:1708–13.
8. Shafran S. Early initiation of antiretroviral therapy: the current best way to reduce liver-related deaths in HIV/hepatitis C virus-coinfected patients. J Acquir Immune Defic Syndr 2007;44:551–6.

9. Blanco F, Barreiro P, Ryan P, et al. Risk factors for advanced liver fibrosis in HIV-infected individuals: role of antiretroviral drugs and insulin resistance. J Viral Hepat 2011;18:11–6.

10. Soriano V, Puoti M, Garcia-Gascó P, et al. Antiretroviral drugs and liver injury. AIDS 2008;22:1–13.

11. Nuñez M. Clinical syndromes and consequences of antiretroviral-related hepatotoxicity. Hepatology 2010;52:1143–55.

12. Labarga P, Soriano V, Vispo ME, et al. Hepatotoxicity of antiretroviral drugs is reduced after successful treatment of chronic hepatitis C in HIV-infected patients. J Infect Dis 2007;196:670–6.

13. Dore G, Torriani F, Rodriguez-Torres M, et al. Baseline factors prognostic of sustained virological response in patients with HIV-hepatitis C virus co-infection. AIDS 2007;21:1555–9.

14. Medrano J, Resino S, Vispo E, et al. HCV treatment uptake and changes in the prevalence of HCV genotypes in HIV/HCV-coinfected patients. J Viral Hepat 2011;18:325–30.

15. Poveda E, Vispo E, Barreiro P, et al. Predicted effect of direct acting antivirals in the current HIV-HCV coinfected population in Spain. Antivir Ther 2012;17:571–5.

16. Maida I, Núñez M, González-Lahoz J, et al. Liver transplantation in HIV-HCV co-infected candidates: what is the most appropriate time for evaluation? AIDS Res Hum Retroviruses 2005;21:599–601.

17. Tan-Tam C, Frassetto L, Stock P. Liver and kidney transplantation in HIV-infected patients. AIDS Rev 2009;11:190–204.

18. Jacobson I, McHutchison J, Dusheiko G, et al. Telaprevir for previously untreated chronic hepatitis C virus infection. N Engl J Med 2011;364:2405–16.

19. Hezode C, Forestier N, Dusheiko G, et al. Telaprevir and peginterferon with or without ribavirin for chronic HCV infection. N Engl J Med 2009;360:1839–50.

20. McHutchison J, Manns M, Muir A, et al. Telaprevir for previously treated chronic HCV infection. N Engl J Med 2010;362:1292–303.

21. Marcellin P, Forns X, Goeser T, et al. Telaprevir is effective given every 8 or 12 hours with ribavirin and peginterferon alfa-2a or 2b to patients with chronic hepatitis C. Gastroenterology 2011;140:459–68.

22. Poordad F, McCone J, Bacon B, et al. Boceprevir for untreated chronic HCV genotype 1 infection. N Engl J Med 2011;364:1195–206.

23. Bacon B, Gordon S, Lawitz E, et al. Boceprevir for previously treated chronic HCV genotype 1 infection. N Engl J Med 2011;364:1207–17.

24. Lenz O, Fevery B, Vijgen L, et al. TMC-435 in patients infected with HCV genotype 1 who have failed previous pegylated interferon/ribavirin treatment: virological analyses of the ASPIRE trial. Presented at 47th EASL, Barcelona, April 18–22, 2012 [abstract 9].

25. Chu T, Kulkarni R, Gane E, et al. Effect of IL28B genotype on early viral kinetics during interferon-free treatment of patients with chronic hepatitis C. Gastroenterology 2012;142:790–5.

26. Seden K, Back D, Shoo S. New directly acting antivirals for hepatitis C: potential for interaction with antiretrovirals. J Antimicrob Chemother 2010;65:1079–85.

27. Jiménez-Nácher I, Alvarez E, Morello J, et al. Approaches for understanding and predicting drug interactions in HIV-infected patients. Expert Opin Drug Metab Toxicol 2011;7:457–77.

28. Soriano V, Sherman K, Rockstroh J, et al. Challenges and opportunities for hepatitis C drug development in HIV-hepatitis C virus-co-infected patients. AIDS 2011;25:2197–208.

29. Rallón N, Naggie S, Benito JM, et al. Association of a single nucleotide polymorphism near the interleukin-28B gene with response to hepatitis C therapy in HIV/hepatitis C virus-coinfected patients. AIDS 2010;24:F23–9.
30. Nattermann J, Vogel M, Nischalke H, et al. Genetic variation in IL28B and treatment-induced clearance of hepatitis C virus in HIV-positive patients with acute and chronic hepatitis C. J Infect Dis 2011;203:595–601.
31. Ryan P, Berenguer J, Michelaud D, et al. Insulin resistance is associated with advanced liver fibrosis and high body mass index in HIV/HCV-coinfected patients. J Acquir Immune Defic Syndr 2009;50:109–10.
32. Cacoub P, Carrat F, Bedossa P, et al. Insulin resistance impairs sustained virological response rate to pegylated interferon plus ribavirin in HIV-hepatitis C virus-coinfected patients: HOMAVIC-ANRS HC02 Study. Antivir Ther 2009;14:839–45.
33. Dieterich D, Soriano V, Sherman K, et al. Telaprevir in combination with peginterferon α-2a plus ribavirin for HIV/HCV coinfected patients: SVR12 interim analysis. Presented at 19th CROI. Seattle (WA), March 5–8, 2012 [abstract 56].
34. Mallolas J, Pol S, Rivero A, et al. Boceprevir plus peginterferon/ribavirin for the treatment of HIV-HCV coinfected patients: end of treatment week 48 interim results. Presented at 47th EASL Barcelona, April 18–22, 2012 [abstract 366].
35. Soriano V, Perelson A, Zoulim F. Why different dynamics of selection of drug resistance in HIV, hepatitis B and C viruses? J Antimicrob Chemother 2008;62:1–4.
36. Morsica G, Bagaglio S, Uberti-Foppa C, et al. Detection of hepatitis C mutants with natural resistance to NS3/4A protease inhibitors in HIV/HCV-coinfected individuals treated with antiretroviral therapy. J Acquir Immune Defic Syndr 2009;51:106–8.
37. Plaza Z, Soriano V, González MM, et al. Impact of antiretroviral therapy on the variability of the HCV NS5B polymerase in HIV-HCV coinfected patients. J Antimicrob Chemother 2011;66:2838–42.
38. Soriano V, Vispo E, Labarga P, et al. Viral hepatitis and HIV co-infection. Antiviral Res 2010;85:303–15.
39. Lafeuillade A, Hittinger G, Chadapaud S. Increased mitochondrial toxicity with ribavirin in HIV/HCV coinfection. Lancet 2001;357:280–1.
40. Mauss S, Valenti W, De Pamphilis J, et al. Risk factors for hepatic decompensation in patients with HIV/HCV coinfection and liver cirrhosis during interferon-based therapy. AIDS 2004;38:F21–5.
41. Garcia-Benayas T, Blanco F, Soriano V. Weight loss in HIV-infected patients. N Engl J Med 2002;347:1287–8.
42. Fleischer R, Boxwell D, Sherman K. Nucleoside analogues and mitochondrial toxicity. Clin Infect Dis 2004;38:e79–80.
43. Vispo E, Barreiro P, Pineda JA, et al. Low response to pegylated interferon plus ribavirin in HIV-infected patients with chronic hepatitis C treated with abacavir. Antivir Ther 2008;13:429–37.
44. Mira JA, López-Cortés L, Barreiro P, et al. Efficacy of pegylated interferon plus ribavirin treatment in HIV/hepatitis C virus co-infected patients receiving abacavir plus lamivudine or tenofovir plus either lamivudine or emtricitabine as nucleoside analogue backbone. J Antimicrob Chemother 2008;62:1365–73.
45. Rodríguez-Nóvoa S, Morello J, González M, et al. Increase in serum bilirubin in HIV/hepatitis C virus-coinfected patients on atazanavir therapy following initiation of pegylated interferon and ribavirin. AIDS 2008;22:2535–7.
46. Van Heeswijk R, Vandervoorde A, Boogaerts G, et al. Pharmacokinetic interactions between ARV agents and the investigational HCV protease inhibitor TVR

in healthy volunteers. Presented at 18th CROI. Boston (MA), February 27–March 2, 2011 [abstract 119].

47. Van Heeswijk R, Gysen V, Boogaerts G, et al. The pharmacokinetic interaction between tenofovir disoproxil fumarate and the investigational HCV protease inhibitor telaprevir. Presented at 48th ICAAC. Washington (DC), October 25–28, 2008. p. A-966.

48. Van Heeswijk R, Boogaerts G, de Paepe E, et al. The pharmacokinetic interaction between escitalopram or esomeprazole and telaprevir. Presented at 15th International Workshop on Clinical Pharmacology of Hepatitis Therapy. Boston (MA), June 23–24, 2010 [abstract 76].

49. Van Heeswijk R, Vandevoorde A, Verboven P, et al. The pharmacokinetic interaction between methadone and the investigational HCV protease inhibitor telaprevir. EASL, Berlin, Germany; March 30-April 3, 2011 [abstract 1244]. J Hepatol 2011;54(Suppl):491–2.

50. Ghosal A, Yuan Y, Tong W, et al. Characterisation of human liver enzymes involved in the biotransformation of boceprevir, a hepatitis C virus protease inhibitor. Drug Metab Dispos 2011;39:510–21.

51. Kasserra C, Hughes E, Treitel M, et al. Clinical pharmacology of BOC: metabolism, excretion and drug-drug interactions. Presented at 18th CROI. Boston (MA), February 27–March 2, 2011 [abstract 118].

52. Rong L, Dahari H, Ribeiro R, et al. Rapid emergence of protease inhibitor resistance in hepatitis C virus. Sci Transl Med 2010;2:30–2.

53. Sarrazin C, Zeuzem S. Resistance to direct antiviral agents in patients with hepatitis C virus infection. Gastroenterology 2010;138:447–62.

54. Guedj J, Perelson A. Second-phase HCV RNA decline during telaprevir-based therapy increases with drug effectiveness: implications for treatment duration. Hepatology 2011;53:1801–8.

55. Halfon P, Locarnini S. Hepatitis C virus resistance to protease inhibitors. J Hepatol 2011;55:192–206.

56. Soriano V, Vispo E, Poveda E, et al. Directly acting antivirals against hepatitis C virus. J Antimicrob Chemother 2011;66:1673–86.

57. Kieffer T, Kwong A, Picchio G. Viral resistance to specifically targeted antiviral therapies for hepatitis C (STAT-Cs). J Antimicrob Chemother 2010;65:202–12.

58. Treviño A, de Mendoza C, Parra P, et al. Natural polymorphisms associated with resistance to new antivirals against hepatitis C virus (HCV) in newly diagnosed HIV/HCV-coinfected patients in Spain. Antivir Ther 2011;16:413–6.

59. Trimoulet P, Belzunce C, Faure M, et al. HCV protease variability and anti-HCV protease inhibitor resistance in HIV/HCV-coinfected patients. HIV Med 2011;12:506–9.

60. Miro JM, Castells L, Valdivieso A, et al. Treatment with pegIFN+RBV of 67 HIV+ patients with recurrent HCV infection after liver transplantation. Presented at CROI 2011. Boston (MA), February 27–March 2, 2011 [abstract 964].

61. Garg V, van Heeswiijk R, Eun-Lee J, et al. Effect of telaprevir on the pharmacokinetics of cyclosporine and tacrolimus. Hepatology 2011;54:20–7.

62. Soriano V. A new era for hepatitis C – new diagnostic tools and new weapons. ACS Med Chem Lett, in press.

Future Classes of Hepatitis C Virus Therapeutic Agents

Jennifer Y. Chen, MD, Raymond T. Chung, MD*

KEYWORDS

- Hepatitis C virus • Antiviral therapeutics • Direct-acting antivirals
- Host-targeted agents

KEY POINTS

- More than 170 million people are infected with chronic HCV, which remains the leading indication for liver transplantation worldwide.
- Recent advances in the understanding of HCV molecular virology have led to the development of novel antiviral therapeutics.
- The HCV life cycle consists of several key steps, including polypeptide cleavage and viral replication, which represent important targets for viral eradication.
- Direct-acting antivirals are designed to inhibit viral targets, and include NS3/4A serine protease inhibitors, NS5B RNA-dependent RNA polymerase inhibitors, and NS5A inhibitors.
- Host-targeted antivirals block host factors that are used by the virus for its own life cycle, and include cyclophilin A inhibitors, miRNA122 inhibitors, and inhibitors of cholesterol biosynthesis.
- The development of agents in multiple classes has led to the promise of shorter therapy duration, an improved side effect profile, interferon-sparing regimens, and higher rates of cure.

INTRODUCTION

More than 170 million people are infected with hepatitis C virus (HCV), which is responsible for approximately 350,000 deaths per year.[1] Of those infected with HCV, up to 80% develop chronic infection, which frequently progresses to cirrhosis, hepatocellular carcinoma, and death.[2,3]

Cure of HCV, or achievement of sustained virologic response (SVR), defined as an undetectable serum HCV RNA measured 24 weeks after the end of treatment, is associated with reduction in the risk of liver-related complications.[4,5] For the past two

GI Unit, Massachusetts General Hospital, GRJ724, 55 Fruit Street, Boston, MA 02114, USA
* Corresponding author.
E-mail address: rtchung@partners.org

Infect Dis Clin N Am 26 (2012) 949–966
http://dx.doi.org/10.1016/j.idc.2012.08.003
0891-5520/12/$ – see front matter Published by Elsevier Inc.

decades, treatment of HCV has centered on the use of pegylated interferon (IFN)-α (peginterferon-α [PEG]) in combination with ribavirin (RBV). Therapy with PEG/RBV has produced overall SVR rates of 54% to 56%, with a rate of 45% to 50% in patients with HCV genotype (GT) 1 (the most common genotype of HCV) and a rate of 80% in patients with HCV GT2 or GT3.[6–8] Long-term follow-up studies have revealed that a SVR is maintained indefinitely and corresponds clinically with cure.[9–11]

However, HCV treatment is associated with numerous side effects, which have led to lack of adherence and premature treatment discontinuation. More specifically, PEG-α is associated with flulike symptoms, cytopenia, autoimmunity, and depression, and RBV causes hemolysis. This multitude of side effects, numerous absolute and relative contraindications, and the less than 50% cure rate achieved among patients with HCV GT1 have limited the real-world effectiveness of PEG and RBV. Most of the 4 million persons in the United States who are infected with HCV have never been treated, let alone cured.

For the first time since the discovery of HCV, recent advances in understanding of the molecular characteristics of the virus have led to the development of novel antiviral therapeutics. Direct-acting antivirals (DAAs) are designed to inhibit viral targets, whereas host-targeted antivirals block host factors that are used by the virus for its own life cycle. In 2011, the first DAAs, telaprevir (TPV) and boceprevir (BOC), were approved by the US Food and Drug Administration (FDA) and the European Medicines Agency for the treatment of chronic HCV GT1 infection, representing an important milestone in HCV therapy. Moreover, the rapid development of agents in multiple classes has led to the promise of shorter therapy duration, an improved side effect profile, and eventually IFN-sparing regimens. This article reviews novel HCV therapeutics in development, including mechanism of action, efficacy, and adverse effects.

HCV VIROLOGY AND LIFE CYCLE

The development of in vitro HCV replication models has greatly increased the understanding of viral structure, entry, replication, and host factors used for virus propagation.[12,13] These advances have enabled the discovery of new strategies aimed at interrupting key steps in the HCV life cycle.

Within the family Flaviviridae, HCV is a linear, positive-sense, single-stranded RNA virus with a 9.6-kb genome. The HCV genome contains an open reading frame that encodes a single polypeptide of approximately 3000 amino acids.

HCV enters hepatocytes through endocytosis and uncoats in a pH-dependent fashion (**Fig. 1**).[14] After uncoating, the positive-sense strand RNA within the virion is used as a template for cytoplasmic translation into the single polypeptide. The polypeptide is cleaved by host and viral proteases, including NS3/4a protease, into 10 proteins: three structural proteins (core, E1, and E2), and seven nonstructural (NS) proteins (p7, NS2, NS3, NS4A, NS4B, NS5A, and NS5B) (**Fig. 1**). Viral replication occurs at an endoplasmic reticulum membrane-derived replication complex, which includes the nonstructural proteins NS4B and NS5A.

Through the activity of the NS5B RNA-dependent RNA polymerase (RdRp) and the NS3 helicase, positive-sense RNA strands are copied into negative-antisense strands in a cyclophilin A– and microRNA-122–dependent fashion. The negative-antisense strands act as a replicative intermediate for copies of positive-sense RNA strands.

Newly produced viral RNA genomes are then encapsidated, and are released by the host plasma membrane. Viral secretion occurs in association with very-low-density lipoproteins, through a process that remains incompletely understood.

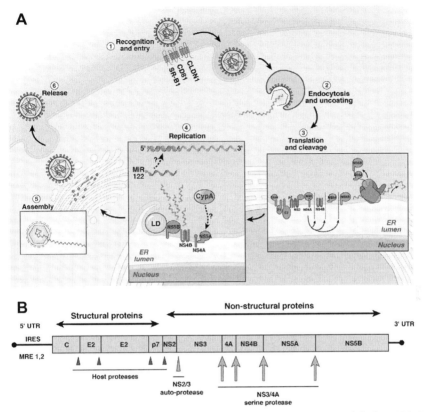

Fig. 1. HCV viral life cycle, HCV polypeptide structure, and cleavage sites. (*A*) The HCV viral life cycle. The virus circulates as a highly lipidated lipoviral particle (LVP). Once internalized, the viral genome is uncoated, revealing the naked viral RNA and viral nucleocapsid. The viral RNA is translated by host ribosomes into the viral polypeptide (*step 3*), which is then cleaved by a combination of host and viral proteases into the 10 viral proteins. Replication occurs at an endoplasmic reticulum membrane-derived replication complex (the membranous web), which includes the lipid droplet (LD) and nonstructural viral proteins NS4A and NS5B (*step 4*). Viral replication is also dependent on the participation of key host factors, which include miR-122 and cyclophilin A (CypA). The newly synthesized viral RNA is assembled into new LVP by the Golgi apparatus and subsequently released by the cell (*steps 5 and 6*). (*B*) HCV viral genome. The viral genome is a positive-sense, single-stranded RNA genome. The 5′ untranslated region (UTR) contains two important domains. The internal ribosome entry site (IRES) directs translation in a cap-independent manner. The 5 = UTR also contains two recognition sites by miR-122 that are critical for viral replication. After translation, a single viral polypeptide is generated. The structural proteins are cleaved by host proteases. The NS2/3 autoprotease cleaves the NS2-NS3 junction. The NS3/4A protease initially serves as an autoprotease and separates NS3-NS4A, but then subsequently cleaves the remaining nonstructural proteins.

The genetic variation of HCV cannot be underestimated. There are six known major genotypes and more than 100 subtypes of HCV. Moreover, the virus produces approximately 10 infectious virions each day in an infected adult, and the error-prone RdRp has no proofreading capability, resulting in a mutation rate of 10^{-4} per nucleotide.[15] The risk for development of resistance poses a significant challenge to the development of novel HCV therapeutics.

DIRECT-ACTING ANTIVIRALS
NS3/4A Serine Protease Inhibitors

Discovery of the NS3/4A crystal structure, in conjunction with mutagenesis studies, has enabled the development of multiple NS3/4A serine protease inhibitors (PIs). Because the protease has a shallow peptide-binding groove, few molecules were identified that blocked NS3/4A activity. Subsequently, peptidomimetic NS3/4A inhibitors were developed, which inhibit enzymatic activity by mimicking the cleavage end product of the proteolytic reaction.

The first drugs in this class approved by the FDA, TPV and BOC, are structurally similar linear molecules that are primarily active against GT1 HCV. TPV and BOC are recommended for use in combination with PEG and RBV. Overall, the efficacy of TPV and BOC seem similar, and are associated with a significant increase in SVR rates in treatment-naive and treatment-experienced subjects with GT1 infection.[16–20] However, TPV and BOC have a low barrier to resistance[21–23]; variable activity against genotypes other than GT1; adverse side effects including rash and anemia; and numerous drug-drug interactions, particularly with drugs metabolized principally by CYP3A4 of the cytochrome P-450 pathway.

Additional inhibitors of the NS3/4A serine protease are in clinical development and can be divided into two categories according to their structure. Linear ketoamide derivates (eg, TPV and BOC) interact with the catalytic site and lead to reversible, covalent inhibition. Macrocyclic inhibitors block the catalytic site by a reversible, noncovalent mechanism, and have a potentially more favorable resistance profile than most linear PIs.[24,25]

BI 201335 is a linear tripeptide PI that has been studied in treatment-naive patients and treatment-experienced patients in two phase IIb trials, SILEN-C1 and SILEN-C2, respectively.[26,27] In the SILEN-C1 study, the addition of BI 201335 dosed at 240 mg daily to PEG/RBV was associated with an increased SVR rate compared with standard of care (SOC; PEG/RBV combination therapy) among treatment-naive patients with GT1: 73% to 83% versus 56%, respectively.[26] In the SILEN-C2 study, BI 201335 was studied in combination with PEG/RBV among prior partial and null responders with GT1 HCV.[27] Rates of SVR were 27% to 41%, which were lower than those observed among treatment-experienced patients who received TPV and BOC in prior trials.[20,28] Furthermore, BI 201335 has been studied as part of an IFN-sparing regimen. Preliminary data from SOUND-C2, a phase IIb trial, revealed an SVR rate of 68% among treatment-naive GT1 patients who received BI 201335 in combination with BI 207127 (a nonnucleoside polymerase inhibitor) and RBV.[29] These data illustrate the efficacy and tolerability of an all-oral combination regimen that includes drugs with different viral targets. Advantages of BI 201335 include its once-daily dosing. Side effects include jaundice, rash, nausea, vomiting, and diarrhea.

TMC-435 is a macrocyclic inhibitor whose improved pharmacokinetic properties, including a 40-hour half-life, allow once-daily dosing.[30] It has antiviral effects against HCV GT1, GT2, GT5, and GT6, but limited efficacy against GT3. A phase IIb study revealed an increased efficacy of TMC-435 in combination with PEG/RBV: more than 90% of patients given TMC-based therapy achieved rapid virologic response and early virologic response (EVR), and rates of SVR were 75% to 85%.[31,32] Side effects of TMC-435 include asymptomatic hyperbilirubinemia. Data suggest an improved resistance profile compared with the linear PI inhibitors.[33]

Danoprevir (ITMN-191/RG7227) is a macrocyclic PI with high specificity and anti-viral efficacy against GT1 HCV, and is dosed two to three times daily.[34] Results from ATLAS, a phase IIB study, revealed that danoprevir in combination with PEG-RBV was associated with SVR rates of 68% to 85%, compared with 42% among those who received SOC.[35] Danoprevir is generally well-tolerated, but associated with increased risk of neutropenia and elevation in alanine aminotransferase. The addition of ritonavir reduces overall systemic exposure to danoprevir (ie, area under the curve and Cmax) than with danoprevir alone while maintaining potency against HCV. The combination, along with PEG and RBV, has been shown to suppress HCV without increasing levels of aminotransferases.[36]

Several other PIs are in clinical development (**Table 1**), including vaniprevir (MK-7009), asunaprevir (BMS-650032), ABT-450, GS-9451, and GS-9256. In addition, MK-5172 has demonstrated potent activity against many of the first-generation PI resistance-associated variants in biochemical assays, and has broad genotypic activity.[37,38]

As with TPV and BOC, a major limitation of PIs has been the rapid development of resistant variants of HCV. When given as monotherapy, PIs exert selective pressure on the population and allow resistant variants to become the dominant viral species. Amino acid changes primarily occur in the NS3 protease catalytic domain and prevent binding of the peptidomimetic inhibitor. However, in vitro studies have demonstrated that HCV variants that are resistant to PIs remain susceptible to other antiviral agents, suggesting the importance of combination therapy with agents from different antiviral classes.

NS5B RdRp Inhibitors

The HCV NS5B protein is an RdRp, which plays a pivotal role in viral replication. The protein has a three-dimensional, right-handed motif in which the palm is the active site of polymerase activity and chain elongation, the thumb plays a significant role in initiation of RNA synthesis, and the fingers and thumb encircle the active site (**Fig. 2**).[39]

Inhibitors of the HCV RdRp are divided into two groups: nucleos(t)ide inhibitors (NIs) and nonnucleoside inhibitors (NNIs). NIs bind to the NS5B active site; compete with nucleotide triphosphates for incorporation into nascent HCV RNA; and once incorporated, prevent chain elongation. Because NIs are already phosphorylated and bypass host phosphorylation steps, they are able to achieve high levels of nucleotide triphosphate in the liver. NNIs bind to one of at least three allosteric pockets outside the active site, and induce a conformational change in the active site that blocks chain elongation.

Nucleos(t)ide Inhibitors

NIs have shown in vitro potency against multiple HCV genotypes, and offer a particularly high barrier to the development of viral resistance because the NS5B active site is intolerant to amino acid substitutions. Thus, active site NS5B mutations that confer resistance to this antiviral class are also more likely to inhibit RdRp activity, rending the mutant virus less "fit" compared with wild-type virus. Cell culture experiments have confirmed that nucleos(t)ide analogues are less likely to select for resistance mutations than NNIs and PIs.

PSI-7977 is a uridine NI administered once daily, and has been studied in several phase II trials. The PROTON study reported SVR rates of 88% to 91% among treatment-naive HCV GTI patients who received PSI-7977 plus PEG-RBV.[40] Of note, the high barrier to resistance of PSI-7977 was shown in this study: no virologic

Table 1
NS3/4A serine protease inhibitors in advanced clinical testing

Drug	Current Phase	Class	Genotype	Dosing	Clinical Data (If Available)[a]	Adverse Effects/Notes
Telaprevir	FDA approved	Linear	1 (2,5,6)	3/day	SVR: 69%–75% (1) SVR (SOC): 44%	Rash, anemia, pruritus
Boceprevir	FDA approved	Linear	1 (2,5,6)	3/day	SVR: 63%–66% (2) SVR (SOC): 40%	Anemia, dysgeusia
TMC-435	Phase 3	Macrocyclic	1 (2,5,6)	1/day	SVR: 75%–85% (3) SVR (SOC): 65%	Elevated bilirubin
BI 201335	Phase 3	Linear tripeptide	1	1/day	SVR: 73%–83% (4) SVR (SOC): 56%	Nausea, diarrhea, jaundice, rash
Narlaprevir	Phase 2	Linear	1	1/day	SVR24: 70%–85% (5) SVR24 (SOC): 28%	Used with ritonavir; fatigue, myalgias
ACH-1625	Phase 2	Linear	1	1/day	RVR: 75%–81% RVR (SOC): 20% (6)	Headache, fatigue, nausea
Danoprevir	Phase 2	Macrocyclic	1	2/day	SVR24: 68%–85% (7) SVR24 (SOC): 42%	ALT elevation decreased when used with ritonavir
Vaniprevir	Phase 2	Macrocyclic	1	2/day	SVR: 61%–84% (8) SVR (SOC): 63%	Headache, nausea, vomiting
ABT-450	Phase 2	Acrylsulfonamide	1	1/day	cEVR: 92% cEVR (SOC): 18% (9)	Used with ritonavir; headache, pruritus
BMS-650032	Phase 2	Active site	1,4	2/day	cEVR: 75%–91.7% (10) cEVR (SOC): 0%	ALT elevation at higher doses
GS-9256	Phase 2	Macrocyclic	1	2/day	cEVR: 100% (11) [b]	Used with tegobuvir
MK-5172	Phase 2	Macrocyclic	1 (2,3,4,5,6)	1/day	75% of GT1 and 38% of GT3 achieved HCV RNA levels below the limit of quantitation with 7 days of monotherapy (12)	Headache, pruritus, nausea, fatigue; pan-genotypic, low cross-resistance (13)
GS-9451	Phase 2	Macrocyclic	1	1/day	n.a.	

Abbreviations: cEVR, complete early virologic response; RVR, rapid virologic response; SOC, standard of care, peglated-interferon-α plus ribavirin; SVR, sustained virologic response; SVR12, undetectable HCV RNA 12 weeks after completion of therapy.
[a] Data are for genotype 1, combined with SOC peglated interferon-α and ribavirin, unless otherwise indicated.
[b] On quadruple therapy including tegobuvir plus SOC, GS-9246 plus SOC not tested.

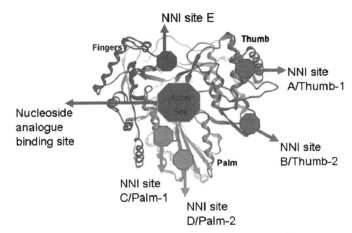

Fig. 2. Nonnucleoside inhibitor (NNI) binding sites on the HCV polymerase. NNIs are allosteric inhibitors of the HCV polymerase. Nucleoside analogs mimic the natural substrate of the HCV polymerase and inhibit it by binding to its active site. *From* McGovern BH, Abu Dayyeh BK, Chung RT. Avoiding therapeutic pitfalls: the rational use of specifically targeted agents against hepatitis C infection. Hepatology 2008;48:1700–12; with permission.

breakthrough was observed during 12 weeks of triple therapy with PSI-7977 at different dosing levels (200 mg and 400 mg once daily). Furthermore, PSI-7977 may be effective in regimens that do not contain PEG. In the ELECTRON study, among 25 treatment-naive patients with GT1 infection who received PSI-7977 and RBV, 88% achieved undetectable HCV RNA 4 weeks after completion of treatment.[41] In the QUANTUM trial, 59% of treatment-naive GT1 patients were HCV RNA undetectable at 4 weeks after treatment with PSI-7977 and RBV.[42] Similarly, among treatment-naive patients with HCV GT2 or GT3 who received 12 weeks of therapy with PSI-7977 and RBV, an SVR of 100% was observed.[43]

Mericitabine (RG7128) is an oral cytosine NI dosed twice daily, and has shown efficacy against GT1, GT2, and GT3 in phase I trials.[44] Results from the JUMP-C study, a phase II trial, highlighted the efficacy of mericitabine in combination with PEG-RBV: at Week 24, 91% of patients who received mericitabine plus PEG-RBV had undetectable HCV RNA compared with 62% who had SOC.[45] In addition, no viral rebound or resistance mutations were observed by Week 12.

NNIs of HCV Polymerase

In contrast to nucelos(t)ide analogues, NNIs have moderate to low antiviral potency and a low barrier to resistance. Because NNIs induce allosteric conformational changes that limit access of the nucleotides to the growing viral RNA chain, mutations that block binding of NNIs do not necessarily reduce viral fitness. Thus, NNIs generally have a low barrier to resistance.

NNIs are categorized according to the site of interaction with the NS5B protein. There are several NNIs in clinical development (**Table 2**), and they include tegobuvir and VX-222. The results of a phase II study of tegobuvir in combination with PEG-RBV were recently reported: similar SVR rates of 56% were observed among treatment-naive chronic GT1 patients who received tegobuvir plus PEG-RBV with those who received SOC.[46] Similarly, when VX-222 was combined with TPV in the ZENITH study among treatment-naive GT1 patients, the results at Week 12 were

Table 2
NS5B nucleos(t)ide inhibitors and nonnucleoside inhibitors

Class(site)	Drug	Current Phase	Genotype	Dosing	Clinical Data (If Available)[a]	Adverse Effects/Notes
Nucleos(t)ide inhibitors						
Active site	Mericitabine	Phase 2b	1–3 (4,5,6)	2/day	SVR12: 91% (14)[b] SVR12 (SOC): 62%	No resistance-related breakthrough
Active site	PSI-7977	Phase 2b	1–3 (4,5,6)	1/day	SVR: 88%–91% EOT (SOC): 50%[c] (15)	Anemia, neutropenia; no viral breakthrough observed
Active site	IDX 184	Phase 2a	(1–6)	1–2/day	RVR: 63%–73% (16)	Anemia, nausea
Nonnucleoside inhibitors						
Thumb Domain 2	Filibuvir	Phase 2b	1	2/day	SVR12: 30%–50% (17) SVR12 (SOC): 50%	High rates of relapse observed
Palm Domain 2	Tegobuvir	Phase 2b	1	2/day	SVR: 56% SVR (SOC): 56% (18)	No significant difference from SOC
Palm Domain 1	Setrobuvir (ANA-598)	Phase 2b	1	2/day	cEVR: 78% cEVR (SOC): 56% (19)	Rash more common at higher doses
Palm Domain 1	ABT-072	Phase 2a	1	1/day	EVR: 70% (20) EVR (SOC): 18%	Unfavorable IL28B genotype associated with failure to achieve cEVR
Palm Domain 1	ABT-333	Phase 2a	1	2/day	EVR: 75% (21) EVR (SOC): 18%	Rash, photosensitivity
Thumb Domain 1	BI 207127	Phase 2a	1	3/day	RVR: 100% (22)[d]	Combined with RBV, and BI 201335 Headache, nausea, pruritus
Thumb Domain 2	VX-222	Phase 2	1	1/day	SVR12: 83%–90% (23)[d]	Fatigue, rash, anemia, pruritus
Palm Domain 2	IDX-375	Phase 2	1	1x/d	n.a.	n.a.

Abbreviations: cEVR, complete early virologic response; RVR, rapid virologic response; SOC, standard of care, pegylated-interferon-α plus ribavirin; SVR, sustained virologic response; SVR12, undetectable HCV RNA 12 weeks after completion of therapy.

[a] Data are for genotype 1, combined with SOC pegylated interferon-α and ribavirin, unless otherwise indicated.
[b] SVR12 based on subset who achieved RVR. SOC data not yet available.
[c] Genotypes 1 SVR (SOC) data pending. 100% SVR was observed in genotype 2/3 patients receiving PSI-7977 and RBV only (21).
[d] No SOC arm for comparison.

disappointing, with 17% to 31% virologic breakthrough rates.[47] However, quadruple therapy consisting of VX-222, TPV, PEG, and RBV seemed to be more effective in the study, with 83% to 90% achieving an undetectable HCV RNA at Week 12.

NS5A Inhibitors

In addition to direct antiviral therapy targeting the NS3/4A serine protease and NS5B RdRp, novel therapeutics have been developed to inhibit the NS5A protein. The NS5A protein is important for viral replication and for the assembly of virions, and is thought to impair the innate immune response, but the precise mechanisms have yet to be characterized.[48–51] The protein consists of three domains: domain I contains an amphipathic domain important for membrane attachment; domain II is thought to have interaction sites for cyclophilin; and domain III is involved in viral assembly.[52]

Daclatasvir (BMS-790052) is an oral NS5A inhibitor with potent in vitro activity. It seems to bind complement domain I of NS5A, and has in vitro activity against all six major viral genotypes, although its in vivo activity against GT2 to GT6 has not yet been demonstrated. A phase II study of daclatasvir revealed high efficacy in treatment-naive GT1 patients treated with this drug combined with PEG-RBV, with SVR12 rates of 83% to 92%.[53] When studied in combination with GS-7977 (NS5B inhibitor) in a phase IIa trial, the once-daily, IFN-free combination therapy demonstrated a 100% response rate at posttreatment Week 4 (SVR4) in treatment-naive patients with GT1 infection.[54]

Moreover, daclatasvir has been studied among patients with GT1 who had not responded to or were intolerant to prior therapy with PEG-RBV: dual therapy with daclatasvir and asunaprevir (an NS3 PI) was associated with an overall 77% SVR rate at 24 weeks.[55] These findings demonstrate that alternatives to IFN-based regimens are feasible and can cure even the most difficult-to-treat patients.

Additional NS5A inhibitors in clinical development include ABT 627 and GS-5885.

ALTERNATE IFNS

The type I IFN-α is a cytokine that induces hundreds of genes that collectively generate an antiviral state, and has been a cornerstone of HCV treatment. In 2009, the identification of the association between possession of single nucleotide polymorphisms near the *IL28B* gene locus on chromosome 19 and HCV clearance has had widespread implications on the understanding of the pathogenesis of HCV and potential therapeutic options, including antiviral drug development. Host *IL28B* genotype has been shown to be an important predictor of SVR after treatment with IFN-based regimens[56,57] and even IFN-sparing regimens.[58] The mechanism for the contribution of *IL28B* genotype to regimens that do not include IFN is unclear, but suggests a host innate component contributes to SVR induced by DAA therapy.

The *IL28B* gene encodes IFN-λ3, a type-3 IFN (along with IFN-λ1 and IFN-λ2). In contrast to IFN-α, type 3 IFNs bear more semblance to interleukin-10 in structure, and signal through a heterodimeric receptor (IFN-λR and interleukin-10R).[59–61] After receptor binding, IFN-λ shares the Janus kinase-signal transducer and activator of transcription signaling pathway with IFN-α and has anti-HCV effects.[62,63]

Type 3 IFNs are attractive therapeutic targets. IFN-λ1 and the IFN-λ1 receptor are expressed at high levels by hepatocytes, but not all tissues.[64] This limited distribution of the IFN-λ1 receptor offers the potential for a more targeted delivery of IFN therapy with decreased systemic toxicity. In a phase Ib study, PEG IFN-λ1 inhibited HCV without significant toxicity.[65] In the phase IIb EMERGE study of treatment-naive patients with HCV GT1, PEG IFN-λ1 plus RBV produced a complete EVR in

30% patients compared with 28% of patients who received PEG IFN-α plus RBV.[66] Although delivered as a weekly subcutaneous injection, similar to PEG IFN-α, there were generally fewer side effects, such as flu-like complaints and cytopenia, and fewer dose reductions among those who received PEG IFN-λ1 and RBV.

HOST-TARGETED AGENTS

An additional approach to HCV therapy includes targeting host proteins used by the virus for its own life cycle. Novel therapeutics within this category include cyclophilin inhibitors, miRNA122 inhibitors, and 3-hydroxy-3-methylglutaryl (HMG) coenzyme A (CoA) reductase inhibitors.

Cyclophilin A Inhibitors

The cellular protein cyclophilin A is required as part of the HCV replication complex, and seems to modulate NS5A function by unclear mechanisms.[67,68] Cyclophilins were identified as therapeutic targets after cyclosporine, an inhibitor to cyclophilin, was found to suppress HCV in vitro and in vivo.[69] However, because cyclosporine also inhibits calcineurin, it exerts immunosuppressive effects that limit its use as anti-HCV therapy. Additional compounds that inhibit cyclophilin but not calcineurin are in clinical development, and include alisporivir and SCY-635.

Alisporivir (DEB025) blocks the isomerase activity of cyclophilin A, preventing the interaction between NS5A and cyclophilin A, and is active against GT1 to GT4.[67,70–72] A phase IIb study, ESSENTIAL, compared alisporivir in combination with PEG-RBV with SOC in treatment-naive patients with HCV GT1.[73] There was a significantly higher rate of SVR among those who received 48 weeks of alisporivir-based triple therapy compared with SOC (76% vs 55%, respectively); however, there was no statistical difference in SVR rate between those who received alisporivir-based therapy for 24 weeks or response-guided alisporivir therapy compared with SOC (53%, 69%, and 55%, respectively). Alisporivir has also been studied in combination with RBV (without PEG) among treatment-naive patients with GT2 or GT3 infection: at posttreatment Week 12, SVR rates of greater than 80% were observed.[74] The FDA has placed alisporivir on clinical hold because of pancreatitis experienced by several patients who received alisporivir in combination with PEG-RBV.

Preliminary studies suggest that cyclophilin inhibitors in general have a high barrier to resistance, and the resistant variants that do occur remain susceptible to DAAs.

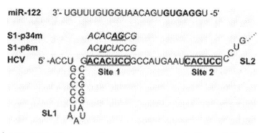

Fig. 3. Sequence of miR-122. Above is shown a representation of the two miR-122–binding sites, S1 and S2, located between stem-loop (SL) 1 and 2 in the 5′ nontranslated region (5′UTR) of the HCV genome. miR122 interacts with two conserved sites, which contain overlapping *cis*-acting signals involved in promoting translation of the virus. (*From* Jangra RK, Yi M, Lemon SM, et al. Regulation of hepatitis C virus translation and infectious virus production by the microRNA miR-122. J Virol 2010;84(13):6615–25; with permission.)

Table 3
Classes of HCV antiviral agents

Class	Potency	Barrier to Resistance	Comments
Protease inhibitors	High	Low	Linear and macrocyclic inhibitors with some cross-resistance
NS5B Nucleos(t)ide inhibitors	Moderate to high	High	Activity across genotypes
NS5B Nonnucleoside inhibitors	Low to moderate	Low	Several allosteric active sites and targets; variable resistance patterns, might be combined
NS5A inhibitors	Moderate to high	Low	NS5A has pleiotropic effects
Cyclophilin inhibitors	Moderate	High	Activity across genotypes
miR122 antagomir	Moderate	High	In early development

miRNA122 Inhibitors

MicroRNAs are short, noncoding RNAs that control gene expression after transcription and are involved in translational repression.[75,76] MicroRNA-122 is the most abundant microRNA found in hepatocytes, and interacts with the HCV genome to promote viral replication (**Fig. 3**).[77–79]

Miravirsen (SPC-3649) is a locked nucleic acid developed to inhibit miR122, and is administered subcutaneously once weekly. It has a high genetic barrier to resistance because it targets host rather than viral RNA, and has potential pangenotypic activity. In a phase II study among treatment-naive GT1 patients, miravirsen monotherapy yielded a mean two to three log HCV RNA reduction from baseline that persisted for weeks beyond treatment and was well-tolerated.[80]

HMG CoA Reductase Inhibitors

HCV replication seems to rely on host cholesterol biosynthetic pathways, in particular with the mevalonate pathway.[81] The HMG CoA reductase and synthase enzymes are involved in HCV replication,[82,83] and inhibitors of HMG CoA reductase (statins) have antiviral effects in vitro [84,85] but limited antiviral effects in vivo.

When given as monotherapy, statins have not been effective against HCV[82]; however, when given in combination with PEG IFN and RBV among treatment-naive patients with GT1 infection, they increased EVR and SVR rates (76% and 64%, respectively).[86]

SUMMARY

Improved understanding of the HCV life cycle and virus-host interactions has led to the development of novel antiviral agents that will significantly expand options for the management of HCV. The addition of two FDA-approved PIs, TPV and BOC, to the SOC regimen has already improved outcomes for patients with HCV GT1 infection.

Moreover, the development of additional classes of antiviral therapeutics, including NS5B RdRp inhibitors, NS5A inhibitors, alternate IFNs, cyclophilin antagonists, and miR122 inhibitors, provides a unique opportunity to redefine the paradigm for the treatment of HCV (**Table 3**). With a rapidly expanding selection of potent agents, it is of critical importance to determine which combination of antiviral drugs provides the most favorable resistance profile with the least toxicity. A multitude of clinical trials is under way to test combinations of agents from distinct antiviral classes with nonoverlapping resistance profiles. Regimens of all-oral DAA have shown efficacy and tolerability in preliminary studies, including among patients who did not respond to prior therapy.[55] Furthermore, improved understanding of the influence of *ILB28* genotype on viral kinetics in response to combination DAA may allow for a more personalized approach to HCV therapy.

With the myriad of anti-HCV therapeutics in the development pipeline, clinicians are firmly on the cusp of a new era. For the first time in 20 years, patients with chronic HCV will soon have access to oral combination therapy associated with a high resistance profile, decreased toxicity, and most importantly, higher rates of cure.

GLOSSARY

- Rapid virologic response (RVR): negative HCV RNA after 4 weeks of treatment
- Early virologic response (EVR): at least a two log reduction in HCV RNA or undetectable HCV RNA after 12 weeks of treatment
  - Complete early virologic response (cEVR): undetectable HCV RNA after 12 weeks of treatment
  - Partial early virologic response (pEVR): at least a two log reduction in HCV RNA, but HCV RNA is detectable after 12 weeks of treatment
- Extended rapid virologic response (eRVR): HCV RNA undetectable at Weeks 4 and 12
- End of treatment response: undetectable HCV RNA at the end of treatment
- Sustained virologic response (SVR): an undetectable serum HCV RNA measured by polymerase chain reaction 24 weeks after the end of treatment.
- Partial responders: patients who achieved a two log reduction in HCV RNA after 12 weeks of treatment but did not achieve an end of treatment response
- Null responders: patients who did not achieve a two log drop in HCV RNA by Week 12 of treatment
- Prior relapsers: patients who achieved an undetectable HCV RNA at the end of treatment but did not achieve a sustained virologic response

REFERENCES

1. Hatzakis A, Wait S, Bruix J, et al. The state of hepatitis B and C in Europe: report from the hepatitis B and C summit conference. J Viral Hepat 2011;18(Suppl 1): 1–16.
2. Page K, Hahn JA, Evans J, et al. Acute hepatitis C virus infection in young adult injection drug users: a prospective study of incident infection, resolution, and reinfection. J Infect Dis 2009;200(8):1216–26.
3. Wang CC, Krantz E, Klarquist J, et al. Acute hepatitis C in a contemporary US cohort: modes of acquisition and factors influencing viral clearance. J Infect Dis 2007;196(10):1474–82.
4. Poynard T, McHutchison J, Manns M, et al. Impact of pegylated interferon alfa-2b and ribavirin on liver fibrosis in patients with chronic hepatitis C. Gastroenterology 2002;122(5):1303–13.
5. Morgan TR, Ghany MG, Kim HY, et al. Outcome of sustained virological responders with histologically advanced chronic hepatitis C. Hepatology 2010; 52(3):833–44.
6. Manns MP, McHutchison JG, Gordon SC, et al. Peginterferon alfa-2b plus ribavirin compared with interferon alfa-2b plus ribavirin for initial treatment of chronic hepatitis C: a randomised trial. Lancet 2001;358(9286):958–65.

7. Fried MW, Shiffman ML, Reddy KR, et al. Peginterferon alfa-2a plus ribavirin for chronic hepatitis C virus infection. N Engl J Med 2002;347(13):975–82.
8. Hadziyannis SJ, Sette H Jr, Morgan TR, et al. Peginterferon-alpha2a and ribavirin combination therapy in chronic hepatitis C: a randomized study of treatment duration and ribavirin dose. Ann Intern Med 2004;140(5):346–55.
9. Veldt BJ, Heathcote EJ, Wedemeyer H, et al. Sustained virologic response and clinical outcomes in patients with chronic hepatitis C and advanced fibrosis. Ann Intern Med 2007;147(10):677–84.
10. Swain MG, Lai MY, Shiffman ML, et al. A sustained virologic response is durable in patients with chronic hepatitis C treated with peginterferon alfa-2a and ribavirin. Gastroenterology 2010;139(5):1593–601.
11. Kagawa T, Keeffe EB. Long-term effects of antiviral therapy in patients with chronic hepatitis C. Hepat Res Treat 2010;2010:562578.
12. Wakita T, Pietschmann T, Kato T, et al. Production of infectious hepatitis C virus in tissue culture from a cloned viral genome. Nat Med 2005;11(7):791–6.
13. Lindenbach BD, Meuleman P, Ploss A, et al. Cell culture-grown hepatitis C virus is infectious in vivo and can be recultured in vitro. Proc Natl Acad Sci U S A 2006; 103(10):3805–9.
14. Dubuisson J, Helle F, Cocquerel L. Early steps of the hepatitis C virus life cycle. Cell Microbiol 2008;10(4):821–7.
15. Pawlotsky JM. Hepatitis C virus genetic variability: pathogenic and clinical implications. Clin Liver Dis 2003;7(1):45–66.
16. McHutchison JG, Everson GT, Gordon SC, et al. Telaprevir with peginterferon and ribavirin for chronic HCV genotype 1 infection. N Engl J Med 2009;360(18): 1827–38.
17. McHutchison JG, Manns MP, Muir AJ, et al. Telaprevir for previously treated chronic HCV infection. N Engl J Med 2010;362(14):1292–303.
18. Jacobson IM, McHutchison JG, Dusheiko G, et al. Telaprevir for previously untreated chronic hepatitis C virus infection. N Engl J Med 2011;364(25): 2405–16.
19. Poordad F, McCone J Jr, Bacon BR, et al. Boceprevir for untreated chronic HCV genotype 1 infection. N Engl J Med 2011;364(13):1195–206.
20. Bacon BR, Gordon SC, Lawitz E, et al. Boceprevir for previously treated chronic HCV genotype 1 infection. N Engl J Med 2011;364(13):1207–17.
21. Rong L, Dahari H, Ribeiro RM, et al. Rapid emergence of protease inhibitor resistance in hepatitis C virus. Sci Transl Med 2010;2(30):30ra32.
22. Sarrazin C, Kieffer TL, Bartels D, et al. Dynamic hepatitis C virus genotypic and phenotypic changes in patients treated with the protease inhibitor telaprevir. Gastroenterology 2007;132(5):1767–77.
23. Susser S, Welsch C, Wang Y, et al. Characterization of resistance to the protease inhibitor boceprevir in hepatitis C virus-infected patients. Hepatology 2009;50(6): 1709–18.
24. Ciesek S, von Hahn T, Manns MP. Second-wave protease inhibitors: choosing an heir. Clin Liver Dis 2011;15(3):597–609.
25. Halfon P, Locarnini S. Hepatitis C virus resistance to protease inhibitors. J Hepatol 2011;55(1):192–206.
26. Sulkowski MS, Ferenci P, Emanoil C, et al. SILEN-C1: Early antiviral activity and safety of BI 201335 combined with peginterferon alfa-2a and ribavirin in treatment-naive patients with chronic genotype 1 HCV infection. Presented at the 60th Annual Meeting of the American Association for the Study of Liver Diseases. Boston, (MA), October 30–November 3, 2009.

27. Sulkowski MS, Bourliere M, Bronowicki JP, et al. SILEN-C2: sustained virologic response (SVR) and safety of BI201335 combined with peginterferon alfa-2a and ribavirin (P/R) in chronic HCV genotype-1 patients with non-response to P/R. Presented at the 46th Annual Meeting of the European Association for the Study of the Liver. Berlin (Germany), March 30–April 3, 2011.

28. Zeuzem S, Andreone P, Pol S, et al. Telaprevir for retreatment of HCV infection. N Engl J Med 2011;364(25):2417–28.

29. Zeuzem S, Soriano V, Asselah T, et al. SVR4 and SVR12 with an interferon-free regimen of BI 201335 and BI 207127, +/- ribavirin, in treatment-naive patients with chronic genotype-1 HCV infection: interim results of SOUND-C2. Presented at the 47th Annual Meeting of the European Association for the Study of the Liver. Barcelona (Spain), April 18–22, 2012.

30. Lin TI, Lenz O, Fanning G, et al. In vitro activity and preclinical profile of tmc435350, a potent hepatitis C virus protease inhibitor. Antimicrob Agents Chemother 2009;53(4):1377–85.

31. Fried M, Buti M, Dore GJ, et al. Efficacy and safety of TMC435 in combination with peginterferon α-2a and ribavirin in treatment-naive genotype-1 HCV patients: 24-week interim results from the pillar study. Presented at the 61st Annual Meeting of the American Association for the Study of Liver Diseases. Boston (MA), October 29–November 2, 2010.

32. Fried M, Buti M, Dore GJ, et al. TMC435 in combination with peginterferon and ribavirin in treatment-naive HCV genotype 1 patients: Final analysis of the pillar phase IIb study. Presented at the 62nd Annual Meeting of the American Association for the Study of Liver Diseases. San Francisco (CA), November 4–8, 2011.

33. Lenz O, Verbinnen T, Lin TI, et al. In vitro resistance profile of the hepatitis C virus ns3/4a protease inhibitor tmc435. Antimicrob Agents Chemother 2010;54(5): 1878–87.

34. Forestier N, Larrey D, Guyader D, et al. Treatment of chronic hepatitis C patients with the ns3/4a protease inhibitor danoprevir (itmn-191/rg7227) leads to robust reductions in viral RNA: a phase 1b multiple ascending dose study. J Hepatol 2011;54(6):1130–6.

35. Terrault N, Cooper C, Balar LA, et al. High sustained virologic response (SVR24) rates with response-guided danoprevir (DNV; RG7227) plus PegIFN α-2a (40KD) and ribavirin (P/R) in treatment-naive HCV genotype 1 (G1) patients: results from the ATLAS study. Presented at the 62nd Annual Meeting of the American Association for the Study of Liver Diseases. San Francisco (CA), November 4–8, 2011.

36. Gane EJ, Rouzier R, Stedman C, et al. Antiviral activity, safety, and pharmacokinetics of danoprevir/ritonavir plus peg-IFN alpha-2a/RBV in hepatitis C patients. J Hepatol 2011;55(5):972–9.

37. Graham D, Acosta A, Guo Z, et al. MK-5172, a second generation HCV NS3/4A protease inhibitor is active against common resistance associated variants (RAVs) and exhibits cross-genotype activity. Presented at the 62nd Annual Meeting of the American Association for the Study of Liver Diseases. San Francisco (CA), November 5–8, 2011.

38. Petry AS, Fraser IP, Van Dyck K, et al. Safety and antiviral activity of MK-5172, a next-generation HCV NS3/4a protease inhibitor with a broad HCV genotypic activity spectrum and potent activity against known resistance mutants, in genotype 1 and 3 HCV-infected patients. Presented at the 62nd Annual Meeting of the American Association for the Study of Liver Diseases. San Francisco (CA), November 5–8, 2011.

39. Kukolj G, McGibbon GA, McKercher G, et al. Binding site characterization and resistance to a class of non-nucleoside inhibitors of the hepatitis C virus ns5b polymerase. J Biol Chem 2005;280(47):39260–7.

40. Lawitz E, Lalezari JP, Hassanein T, et al. Once-daily PSI-7977 plus Peg/RBV in treatment-naïve patients with HCV GT1: robust end of treatment response rates are sustained post-treatment. Presented at the 62nd Annual Meeting of the American Association for the Study of Liver Diseases (AASLD 2011). San Francisco, November 4–8. 2011.

41. Gane EJ, Stedman CA, Hyland RH, et al. ELECTRON: once daily PSI-7977 plus RBV in HCV GT1/2/3. Presented at the 47th Annual Meeting of the European Association for the Study of the Liver (EASL). Barcelona (Spain), April 18–22, 2012.

42. EASL 2012: Gilead announces early sustained virologic response rates for GS-7977 plus ribavirin in genotype 1 treatment-naïve hepatitis C patients. 2012. Available at: http://hepatitiscresearchandnewsupdates.blogspot.com/2012/04/easl-2012-gilead-announces-early.html#.T7v6_FlZd8E. Accessed May 5, 2012.

43. Gane EJ, Stedman CA, Hyland RH, et al. PSI-7977: ELECTRON interferon is not required for sustained virologic response in treatment-naïve patients with HCV GT2 or GT3. Presented at the 62nd Annual Meeting of the American Association for the Study of Liver Diseases. San Francisco (CA), November 5–8, 2011.

44. Le Pogam S, Seshaadri A, Ewing A, et al. Rg7128 alone or in combination with pegylated interferon-alpha2a and ribavirin prevents hepatitis C virus (HCV) replication and selection of resistant variants in HCV-infected patients. J Infect Dis 2010;202(10):1510–9.

45. Pockros P, Jensen D, Tsai N, et al. First SVR data with the nucleoside analogue polymerase inhibitor mericitabine (RG7128) combined with peginterferon/ribavirin in treatment-naive HCV G1/4 patients: interim analysis from the JUMP-C trial. Presented at the 46th Annual Meeting of the European Association for the Study of the Liver. Berlin (Germany), March 30–April 3, 2011.

46. Lawitz E, Jacobson I, Godofsky E, et al. A phase 2b trial comparing 24 to 48 weeks treatment with tegobuvir (GS-9190)/PEG/RBV to 48 weeks treatment with PEG/RBV for chronic genotype 1 HCV infection. Presented at the European Association for the Study of the Liver (EASL) 46th Annual Meeting. Berlin (Germany), March 30–April 3, 2011.

47. Di Bisceglie AM, Nelson DR, Gane E, et al. VX-222 with TVR alone or in combination with peginterferon alfa-2a and ribavirin in treatment-naive patients with chronic hepatitis C: ZENITH study interim results. Presented at the 46th Annual Meeting of the European Association for the Study of the Liver. Berlin (Germany), March 30–April 3, 2011.

48. Fridell RA, Qiu D, Valera L, et al. Distinct functions of ns5a in hepatitis C virus RNA replication uncovered by studies with the ns5a inhibitor BMS-790052. J Virol 2011;85(14):7312–20.

49. Ferraris P, Blanchard E, Roingeard P. Ultrastructural and biochemical analyses of hepatitis C virus-associated host cell membranes. J Gen Virol 2010;91(Pt 9):2230–7.

50. Macdonald A, Harris M. Hepatitis C virus ns5a: tales of a promiscuous protein. J Gen Virol 2004;85(Pt 9):2485–502.

51. Lan KH, Lan KL, Lee WP, et al. HCV ns5a inhibits interferon-alpha signaling through suppression of stat1 phosphorylation in hepatocyte-derived cell lines. J Hepatol 2007;46(5):759–67.

52. Gish RG, Meanwell NA. The ns5a replication complex inhibitors: difference makers? Clin Liver Dis 2011;15(3):627–39.

53. Pol S, Ghalib RH, Rustgi VK, et al. First report of SVR12 for a NS5A replication complex inhibitor, BMS-790052, in combination with PeglFNα-2a and RBV: phase IIA trial in treatment-naive HCV genotype 1 subjects. Presented at the 46th Annual Meeting of the European Association for the Study of the Liver (EASL). Berlin, March 30–April 3, 2011.

54. Sulkowski M, Gardiner D, Lawitz E, et al. Potent viral suppression with all-oral combination of daclatasvir (NS5A inhibitor) and GS-7977 (NS5B inhibitor), +/-ribavirin, in treatment-naive patients with chronic HCV GT1, 2, or 3. Presented at the 47th Annual Meeting of the European Association for the Study of the Liver. Barcelona (Spain), April 18–22, 2012.

55. Suzuki F, Ikeda K, Toyota J, et al. Dual oral therapy with the NS5a inhibitor daclatasvir (BMS-790052) and NS3 protease inhibitor asunaprevir BMS-650032) in HCV genotype 1b-infected null responders or ineligible/intolerant to peginterferon/ribavirin. Presented at the 47th Annual Meeting of the European Association for the Study of the Liver. Barcelona (Spain), April 18–22, 2012.

56. Ge D, Fellay J, Thompson AJ, et al. Genetic variation in IL28B predicts hepatitis C treatment-induced viral clearance. Nature 2009;461:399–401.

57. Thompson AJ, Muir AJ, Sulkowski MS, et al. Interleukin-28B polymorphism improves viral kinetics and is the strongest pretreatment predictor of sustained virologic response in genotype 1 hepatitis C virus. Gastroenterology 2010;139: 120–9.

58. Chu TW, Kulkarni R, Gane EJ, et al. Effect of *IL28B* genotype on early viral kinetics during interferon-free treatment of patients with chronic hepatitis C. Gastroenterology 2012;142:790–5.

59. Kotenko SV, Gallagher G, Baurin VV, et al. IFN-lambdas mediate antiviral protection through a distinct class II cytokine receptor complex. Nat Immunol 2003;4(1): 69–77.

60. Sheppard P, Kindsvogel W, Xu W, et al. Il-28, IL-29 and their class II cytokine receptor IL-28R. Nat Immunol 2003;4(1):63–8.

61. Gad HH, Dellgren C, Hamming OJ, et al. Interferon-lambda is functionally an interferon but structurally related to the interleukin-10 family. J Biol Chem 2009; 284(31):20869–75.

62. Zhang L, Jilg N, Shao RX, et al. IL28b inhibits hepatitis C virus replication through the jak-stat pathway. J Hepatol 2011;55(2):289–98.

63. Doyle SE, Schreckhise H, Khuu-Duong K, et al. Interleukin-29 uses a type 1 interferon-like program to promote antiviral responses in human hepatocytes. Hepatology 2006;44(4):896–906.

64. Sommereyns C, Paul S, Staeheli P, et al. IFN-lambda (IFN-lambda) is expressed in a tissue-dependent fashion and primarily acts on epithelial cells in vivo. PLoS Pathog 2008;4(3):e1000017.

65. Muir AJ, Shiffman ML, Zaman A, et al. Phase 1b study of pegylated interferon lambda 1 with or without ribavirin in patients with chronic genotype 1 hepatitis C virus infection. Hepatology 2010;52(3):822–32.

66. Zeuzem S, Arora S, Bacon B, et al. Pegylated interferon-lambda (PegIFN-λ) shows superior viral response with improved safety and tolerability versus PeglFNα-2a in HCV patients (G1/2/3/4): EMERGE phase IIb through week 12. Presented at the 46th Annual Meeting of the European Association for the Study of the Liver. Berlin (Germany), March 30–April 3, 2011.

67. Coelmont L, Hanoulle X, Chatterji U, et al. Deb025 (alisporivir) inhibits hepatitis C virus replication by preventing a cyclophilin A induced cis-trans isomerisation in domain II of ns5a. PLoS One 2010;5(10):e13687.

68. Hanoulle X, Badillo A, Wieruszeski JM, et al. Hepatitis C virus ns5a protein is a substrate for the peptidyl-prolyl cis/trans isomerase activity of cyclophilins A and B. J Biol Chem 2009;284(20):13589–601.

69. Teraoka S, Mishiro S, Ebihara K, et al. Effect of cyclosporine on proliferation of non-A, non-B hepatitis virus. Transplant Proc 1988;20(3 Suppl 3):868–76.

70. Landrieu I, Hanoulle X, Bonachera F, et al. Structural basis for the non-immunosuppressive character of the cyclosporin A analogue debio 025. Biochemistry 2010;49(22):4679–86.

71. Crabbe R, Vuagniaux G, Dumont JM, et al. An evaluation of the cyclophilin inhibitor debio 025 and its potential as a treatment for chronic hepatitis C. Expert Opin Investig Drugs 2009;18(2):211–20.

72. Flisiak R, Feinman SV, Jablkowski M. The cyclophilin inhibitor debio 025 combined with peg ifnalpha2a significantly reduces viral load in treatment-naive hepatitis C patients. Hepatology 2009;49(5):1460–8.

73. Flisiak R, Pawlotsky JM, Crabbé R, et al. Once daily alisporivir (DEB025) plus pegIFNalfa2a/ribavirin results in superior sustained virologic response (SVR24) in chronic hepatitis C genotype 1 treatment naive patients. Presented at the 46th Annual Meeting of the European Association for the Study of the Liver. Berlin (Germany), March 30–April 3, 2011.

74. Pawlotsky JM, Sarin SK, Foster G, et al. Alisporivir plus ribavirin is highly effective as interferon-free or interferon-add-on regimen in previously untreated HCV-GT2 or GT3 patients: SVR12 results from VITAL-1 phase 2b study. Presented at the 47th Annual Meeting of the European Association for the Study of the Liver. Barcelona (Spain), April 18–22, 2012.

75. Guo H, Ingolia NT, Weissman JS, et al. Mammalian micrornas predominantly act to decrease target mRNA levels. Nature 2010;466(7308):835–40.

76. Bartel DP. MicroRNAs: target recognition and regulatory functions. Cell 2009; 136(2):215–33.

77. Jopling CL, Yi M, Lancaster AM, et al. Modulation of hepatitis C virus RNA abundance by a liver-specific microrna. Science 2005;309(5740):1577–81.

78. Jopling CL, Schutz S, Sarnow P. Position-dependent function for a tandem microrna mir-122-binding site located in the hepatitis C virus RNA genome. Cell Host Microbe 2008;4(1):77–85.

79. Jangra RK, Yi M, Lemon SM. Regulation of hepatitis C virus translation and infectious virus production by the microrna mir-122. J Virol 2010;84(13):6615–25.

80. Reesink HW, Janssen HL, Zeuzem S, et al. Final results: randomized, double-blind, placebo-controlled safety, anti-viral proof-of-concept study of miravirsen, an oligonucleotide targeting miR-122, in treatment-naive patients with genotype 1 chronic HCV infection. Presented at the 47th Annual Meeting of the European Association for the Study of the Liver. Barcelona (Spain), April 18–22, 2012.

81. Herker E, Ott M. Unique ties between hepatitis C virus replication and intracellular lipids. Trends Endocrinol Metab 2011;22(6):241–8.

82. Ye J, Wang C, Sumpter R Jr, et al. Disruption of hepatitis C virus RNA replication through inhibition of host protein geranylgeranylation. Proc Natl Acad Sci U S A 2003;100(26):15865–70.

83. Peng LF, Schaefer EA, Maloof N, et al. Ceestatin, a novel small molecule inhibitor of hepatitis C virus replication, inhibits 3-hydroxy-3-methylglutaryl-coenzyme A synthase. J Infect Dis 2011;204(4):609–16.

84. Ikeda M, Abe K, Yamada M, et al. Different anti-hcv profiles of statins and their potential for combination therapy with interferon. Hepatology 2006;44(1): 117–25.

85. O'Leary JG, Chan JL, McMahon CM, et al. Atorvastatin does not exhibit antiviral activity against HCV at conventional doses: a pilot clinical trial. Hepatology 2007; 45(4):895–8.

86. Georgescu EF, Streba L, Teodorescu R, et al. Potential enhancement of both early (EVR) and sustained (SVR) virological response by fluvastatin in chronic hepatitis C treated with standard pegIFN-ribavirin therapy. A pilot study. Presented at the European Association for the Study of the Liver, International Liver Conference, Berlin (Germany), March 30-April 3, 2011.

Hepatitis C Virus Drug Resistance
Implications for Clinical Management

David L. Wyles, MD

KEYWORDS

- Hepatitis C virus • Resistance • Protease inhibitors

KEY POINTS

- The hepatitis C virus life cycle favors rapid resistance selection but not persistence.
- Resistant variants likely pre-exist in all patients.
- Drug-resistant variants are rapidly selected during monotherapy with most direct-acting antivirals.
- Complete cross-resistance exists between currently approved hepatitis C virus protease inhibitors.
- Pre-existing resistant variants do not impact responses to telaprevir or boceprevir therapy in combination with pegylated interferon and ribavirin.

INTRODUCTION

The addition of hepatitis C virus (HCV) NS3 protease inhibitors (PIs) to interferon (IFN)-based regimens has dramatically improved response rates.[1–4] Despite these improvements treatment is now more complex, associated with increased side effects, and has the potential to select resistant variants in those who are not cured. The clinical impact of pre-existing and treatment-selected resistant variants continues to be studied; however, given the rapid uptake of PI use in the community, interim guidance on assessing and interpreting resistance data is necessary. This article discusses the virologic underpinnings for the development of HCV-resistant variants (with a focus on telaprevir and boceprevir) and their impact on therapeutic success. Interim guidance on the use of resistance testing and management is provided based on the limited data. Finally, resistance considerations for other classes of inhibitors and the rapidly approaching IFN-free therapeutics regimens are offered.

HEPATITIS C VIROLOGY AND RESISTANCE POTENTIAL

The HCV is a flavivirus and the only member of the genus *Hepacivirus*. It is a single-stranded, positive-sense RNA virus, and typical of most RNA viruses, possesses an

Division of Infectious Diseases, University of California, San Diego, 9500 Gilman Drive, MC 0711, La Jolla, CA 92093, USA
E-mail address: dwyles@ucsd.edu

Infect Dis Clin N Am 26 (2012) 967–978
http://dx.doi.org/10.1016/j.idc.2012.08.005
0891-5520/12/$ – see front matter © 2012 Elsevier Inc. All rights reserved.

RNA polymerase of low fidelity without a proofreading mechanism. The sequence change rate of HCV has been estimated to be in the range of 10^{-3} to 10^{-4} substitutions per site per year, among the highest evolution rates of viruses infecting human.[5–7] Virion production also occurs at an exceedingly high rate in most chronically infected individuals. Viral kinetic studies during IFN therapy suggest that from 10^{11} to 10^{12} virions are produced per day in infected individuals.[8] The combination of error-prone replication with high rates of viral production results in a remarkably diverse virus globally and within an infected individual.[5]

These characteristics also suggest that resistance to direct-acting antivirals, such as the NS3 PIs, pre-exists at low levels in all chronically infected persons before any antiviral therapy. Rong and colleagues[9] used viral kinetics data and mathematical modeling to quantify the likelihood of pre-existing resistant variants. Using conservative estimates for polymerase error rate and viral turnover they demonstrated that all single- and double-nucleotide mutants are generated daily in infected persons. Additionally, a third mutant (or variant) would be rapidly selected within the first day of antiviral therapy. The implications of these findings bear directly on the design of IFN-free HCV antiviral regimens and the risk of resistance development.

VIRAL RESERVOIRS AND THE PERSISTENCE OF RESISTANT VARIANTS

HIV is the prototypical chronic viral infection where resistance to antivirals is of great clinical significance; it is instructive to compare the virus lifecycles of HIV and HCV from a resistance development and persistence perspective. Although both viruses possess error-prone polymerases, the RNA polymerase of HCV displays a higher rate of misincorporation than does HIV-RT.[6,7,10] Virion production is also 100- to 1000-fold higher in those patients with HCV.[8,11] These characteristics, combined with a lack of overlapping reading frames, suggest that the short-term resistance development potential is higher with HCV than HIV. However, the HCV replication cycle, which occurs exclusively in the cytoplasm without a DNA intermediate, does not provide a means by which resistance mutations can be archived.[12] In glaring contrast, rapid turnover of HIV-infected CD4 T-cell provides ample opportunity for infection and propagation of HIV-resistant variants once selected. Additionally, integration of HIV proviral DNA facilitates the creation of archival sequences harboring resistant variants that occasionally result in long-lived, latently infected cells.[13–15]

RESISTANCE TO APPROVED HCV PIS: IN VITRO AND CLINICAL DATA

Resistance to the antiviral activity of boceprevir and telaprevir emerges rapidly in vitro and in subjects exposed to monotherapy.[16,17] Phenotypic resistance is heralded by the selection of viral variants with characteristic amino acid substitutions in the NS3/4A protease that become the predominant viral population shortly after drug exposure. The variants of primary clinical significance include V36M/A, T54A/S, V55A, R155K/T, A156S/T/V, and V170A.[16–19]

During 14 days of telaprevir monotherapy, most subjects had resistant variants detected with population sequencing after completion of dosing; the primary resistance variants in those with low telaprevir exposure were R155K and V36M (often found in combination). As telaprevir exposure increased, variants at position 156 predominated. In line with the exposure data, R155K confers a modest increase in telaprevir EC_{50} in vitro but better preserved replicative capacity. In contrast, mutants at position 156, particularly the A156T/V variants, result in a large fold-change in EC_{50} but also hamper replicative fitness (**Table 1**).[16] Low-dose boceprevir monotherapy studies revealed an overall similar resistance profile, with the exception of the V55A

Table 1
In vitro fold-change in replicon EC_{50} and relative fitness for common clinical telaprevir and boceprevir resistant variants

Resistant Variant	Fold Change EC_{50}		Relative Fitness (%)
	Telaprevir	Boceprevir	
V36M/A	6–10	2–3	45–75
T54A/S	5–10	6–16	65
V55A	3	4–7	35
R155K/T/M/I	5–10	3–7	50–95
A156S	15–20	5–15	35–50
A156T/V	>100	>100	15–30
V170A	3	3–12	23–170
V36M + R155K	>25	10	42

For position with multiple variants fold-change and fitness are described for the variants listed in bold print.
Data from References.[16,17,24,39,40]

and V170A mutants, which were not seen with telaprevir monotherapy.[17] Wild-type virus predominated after monotherapy and the A156T/V variants were not identified, likely reflecting low boceprevir exposure.[17] In vitro the V55A and V170A mutants result in modest fold-change increases in the enzyme IC_{50} and replicon EC_{50} for telaprevir and boceprevir.[17] Taken together in vitro and clinical monotherapy data suggest a low barrier to resistance for telaprevir and boceprevir with overlapping resistance profiles.

PI RESISTANCE WHEN GIVEN IN COMBINATION WITH PEGYLATED IFN AND RIBAVIRIN

Several important concepts regarding PI resistance were elucidated during the phase 2 and 3 studies with boceprevir or telaprevir in combination with pegylated IFN (PEG) and ribavirin (RBV): (1) most subjects failing PI-based HCV therapy have detectable resistance mutations; (2) low-dose RBV or RBV-free treatment regimens result in high rates of virologic breakthrough and resistance development; (3) the presence of baseline resistant variants detectable by population sequencing occurs in approximately 5% of subjects and, in general, does not impact the response to therapy; and (4) after the removal of drug selective pressure, the prevalence of resistant variants decays with an apparent return to pretreatment levels in most subjects within 2 to 3 years.[1,3,20–23]

In phase 2 studies of telaprevir (12 weeks) with PEG and RBV (24 weeks), viral breakthrough occurred in 5% to 7% of treatment-naive subjects and was more common in those with genotype 1a (7%) than 1b (2%).[21,22] Viral relapse after therapy occurred in 10% to 14% of subjects. Resistant variants identified on breakthrough conferred high-level TPV resistance (defined as >25-fold increase in replicon EC_{50}) and segregated by HCV subtype with the V36M + R155K double mutant occurring in 1a and the A156T/V mutant in 1b.[24] Resistant variants seen on failure after exposure to boceprevir were generally similar to those seen with telaprevir, the most frequent (>25%) being V36M, T54S, and R155K.[23] Two variants not described in telaprevir phase 2b clinical studies, V55A and V170A, were seen with moderate frequency (5%–25%).[23]

THE ROLE OF RBV IN THE PREVENTION OF RESISTANCE DEVELOPMENT

The importance of RBV for prevention of PI resistance development was demonstrated in phase 2 trials of telaprevir and boceprevir. In the PROVE2 study a 24% breakthrough and 48% relapse rate was observed among subjects assigned to the telaprevir/PEG/placebo arm.[21] In treatment-experienced patients, RBV-free treatment (24 weeks of telaprevir plus PEG) resulted in a 32% breakthrough and a 53% relapse rate.[20] Similarly, a phase 2b study of boceprevir treatment-naive subjects assigned to a low-dose RBV arm (400–1000 mg) in combination with PEG had high rates of virologic breakthrough and relapse (27% and 22%, respectively).[23] These findings have resulted in the recommendation that boceprevir and telaprevir always be given in combination with both PEG and RBV.[18,19]

DECAY OF RESISTANT VARIANTS AFTER TREATMENT CESSATION

Resistance analyses of non-sustained virologic response (SVR) subjects in phase 3 studies demonstrated that 53% and 74% of non-SVR subjects in boceprevir and telaprevir studies, respectively, had detectable resistant variants by population sequencing.[25,26] As suggested in early studies there was a strong subtype dependence on the frequency and distribution of variants selected. In telaprevir-treated non-SVR subjects 84% of genotype 1a versus 54% of genotype 1b subjects harbored resistant variant after treatment.[25] Subjects with genotype 1a routinely select for V36M and R155K individually or in combination after PI exposure. Genotype 1b subjects exposed to boceprevir select for variants T54A/S (79%) most frequently with V55A (24%), A156S (26%), and V170A (32%) also occurring.[26] Common telaprevir-resistant variants in genotype 1b subjects include T54A (22%), V36A (16%), and A156S/T (13%).[25]

During follow-up after treatment discontinuation, resistant variants were no longer detectable by population sequencing in most subjects; 22% of subjects treated with boceprevir at 6 to 14 months follow-up and 29% treated with telaprevir at 12 months posttreatment continued to have detectable variants.[25,26] Variants that seemed less fit in vitro decayed by population sequencing at a more rapid rate. During long-term follow-up (mean 29 months) of 126 non-SVR subjects resistant variants were no longer detectable in 85% of subjects by population sequencing.[27] In a subset of 20 patients who had wild-type virus by population sequencing, clonal analysis did not indicate an enrichment of resistant variants at low levels (<5%) after PI exposure; both baseline (~80 clones) and posttreatment (~90 clones) samples contained approximately 1% resistant variants.[28] Despite these reassuring data there are no robust clinical trial data, aside from anecdotal reports, on response rates for subjects retreated with a regimen containing an agent to which they previously had selected resistant variants.

BASELINE RESISTANCE VARIANTS AND RESPONSE TO THERAPY

In subjects enrolled in phase 3 trials, pretreatment population sequencing identified predominant resistant variants in 5% to 7% of subject, with the T54S variant being most common.[18,19] Key variants, such as the R155K or A156S/T, are infrequently found (<1% baseline). Overall, the presence of detectable baseline resistant variants did not adversely impact response rates to boceprevir-based triple therapy for HCV.[19]

However, in patients who are poorly IFN responsive, the risk of virologic failure is high among those who harbor key resistant variants at baseline.[19,29] For example, in the REALIZE trail, all five prior null responders who harbored telaprevir-resistant variants (V36M, T54A/S, V55A, or R155K) at baseline experienced virologic failure.

In contrast, only 1 of 11 patients with a history of either partial response or relapse and the same baseline variants experienced virologic failure on telaprevir.[29] A follow-up study using ultradeep sequencing in 15 null responders from the same study, 14 of whom did not have detectable variants by population sequencing at baseline, suggests that identification of additional mutants by deep sequencing adds no additional predictive value in this situation.[30] Similarly data from boceprevir phase 3 trials showed that the combination of less than 1 $\log_{10}$ decrease in HCV RNA during lead-in combined with predominant variants at positions V36M, T54A/S, V55A, or R155K resulted in no SVRs (zero of seven).[19] It must be kept in mind that subjects fitting these criteria account for a very small percentage of the overall population treated with boceprevir or telaprevir in phase 3 studies ($\sim$1%) and thus the use of these findings in the clinic is limited.

HCV RESISTANCE TESTING AND CLINICAL PRACTICE

HIV drug resistance testing is recommended before initiating therapy in treatment-naive individuals and when altering therapy in those experiencing treatment failure.[31] The use of this approach for HIV lies in the significant rate of transmitted drug resistance and the impact of drug resistance mutations on virologic responses to initial or salvage regimens.[32–35] These recommendations are also made possible by the availability of multiple antiretrovirals, which may be chosen in part based on the resistant profile obtained.

A genotypic HCV resistance assay based on NS3/4A sequencing is commercially available (HCV Genosure NS3/4A; LabCorp/Monogram [Monogram Biosciences, Inc., 345 Oyster Point Blvd., South San Francisco, USA]). This population-based sequencing assay is expected to reliably detect resistant variants present in 20% to 25% of the viral population, although resistant variants present in as little as 10% of the population may be detected.[36] Although resistance testing should clearly be part of investigational trials, the impact of HCV genotypic resistance testing in clinical practice is unclear and is not currently recommended. At present the approved HCV PIs have completely overlapping resistance profiles, and baseline resistance variants do not seem to impact treatment responses to PIs in combination with PEG/RBV for most patients. The use of HCV resistance testing may change with the advent of IFN-free combination therapy relying on multiple agents with unique resistance profiles.

RESISTANCE AND OTHER NOVEL HCV ANTIVIRALS

Potent antivirals with several different mechanisms of action have advanced to phase 2 and 3 studies. Key among these inhibitors is next-generation PIs, nucleoside/nucleotide and nonnucleoside NS5B polymerase inhibitors, and NS5A inhibitors. General resistance characteristics of the inhibitor classes are highlighted in **Table 2**.

Despite dramatic increases in efficacy, boceprevir and telaprevir are limited from a pharmacokinetic, side effect, and resistance barrier standpoint. Next-generation PIs, such as TMC-435 and BI-201355, have improved pharmacokinetics facilitating once-daily dosing and higher response rates in combination with PEG/RBV in phase 2b studies (81%–86%).[37,38] Resistance profiles for these compounds overlap with boceprevir and telaprevir at key positions; in particular, variants at arginine 155 (R155K) and alanine 156 (A156T/V) confer resistance to these compounds in vitro.[39,40]

In contrast to the linear ketoamides boceprevir and telaprevir, macrocyclic PIs, such as TMC-435, do not show appreciable increases in replicon EC_{50}s in vitro to variants V36M, T54A/S, A156S, or V170A.[39,40] Mutations at position D168 (D168E/H/A/V) of the protease gene confer moderate to high level resistance (>500-fold for A/V variants)

Table 2
Summary of resistance characteristics for HCV inhibitors classes

Inhibitor Class	Resistance Characteristics
Protease inhibitors	• Low-resistance barrier (increased with later-generation compounds) • Extensive cross-resistance • Resistance barrier variation by subtype (1a <1b) • Pre-existing variants rare
Nonnucleoside polymerase inhibitors	• Lowest resistance barrier • Unique allosteric sites with unique resistance profiles • Pre-existing variants more common
Nucleoside/nucleotide polymerase inhibitors	• Highest resistance barrier • Clinical resistance extremely rare • Pre-existing variants not described
NS5A inhibitors	• Low-resistance barrier • Extensive cross-resistance • Resistance barrier variation by subtype (1a <1b) • Pre-existing variants rare

to the macrocyclic inhibitors but do not result in cross-resistance to telaprevir and boceprevir.[39–41] In clinical trials of macrocylic PIs the R155K variants predominate in those with genotype 1a experiencing virologic failure, whereas variants at position 168 predominate in 1b subjects.[42–44] Ritonavir-boosting, when possible, may improve the resistance barrier of HCV PIs by optimizing pharmacokinetics. During 3-day mono-therapy with ritonavir-boosted ABT-450, a macrocyclic PI, a decrease in selected resistant variants was noted in the 200-mg versus 50-mg groups.[45] Finally, MK-5172 is a "latest-generation" macrocyclic PI that retains activity against the R155K mutant in vitro and was extremely potent in phase 1b studies.[46,47]

NS5B polymerase inhibitors come in two classes. Nucleoside/nucleotide inhibitors (NI) target the active site and act as RNA chain terminators. Nonnucleoside inhibitors (NNI) bind to one of at least four unique allosteric sites and work by inhibiting confor-mational changes in the polymerase necessary for productive RNA replication.[48] NNI targeting a specific allosteric site tend to select for the same resistant variants and display extensive cross-resistance (reviewed in[49]). In addition, allosteric inhibitor binding sites are not highly conserved and viral variants with polymorphisms resulting in resistance to NNI are more prevalent than pre-existing resistant variants to PI or NS5A inhibitors.[50] The prevalence of these variants varies depending on the sensitivity of the methodology used. In a study using population-based sequencing, NNI-resistant variants were found in 2.8% of 507 subjects.[51] However, a smaller study performing a clonal analysis on 13 subjects (80–90 clones per) found that 11 (85%) of 13 harbored baseline variants (1%–5% of the viral population) associated with resis-tance to palm site NNIs.[52] An ultradeep sequencing analysis found baseline resistant variants to NNIs in 22.5% of 89 samples at a threshold of greater than or equal to 0.5%.[50] Polymorphic target sites contributing to modest antiviral potency result in very low barriers to resistance for NNIs as a class.

In contrast to NNIs, NIs target the highly conserved polymerase active site; pre-existing polymorphisms conferring reduced susceptibility to NIs have not been described.[50,52] In vitro resistance to 2′-C-methyl nucleosides can be selected and is associated with the S282T variant, which has poor replicative fitness and confers only a modest increase in EC_{50}.[53–55] Consistent with in vitro resistance data, the S282T variant has rarely been identified after unsuccessful NI treatment in vivo.[56] In recent clinical trials the S282T mutant has not been observed with regimens consisting of GS-7977 plus RBV (with or without PEG) or mericitabine with PEG and RBV; however, additional viral sequencing remains to be completed.[57,58] Although more data are needed, it is clear from in vitro studies and clinical data that HCV NIs possess a very high barrier to resistance making them attractive as components of IFN-free HCV treatment regimens.

BMS-790052 is a potent NS5A inhibitor that has advanced into phase 3 clinical trials with PEG/RBV and offers improved response rates (83% SVR) and once-daily dosing.[59,60] Similar to PIs, resistant variants are rapidly selected and become the predominant population after short-course monotherapy.[61] Variants at positions M28, Q30, L31, and Y93 in genotype 1a and L31 and Y93 in genotype 1b are commonly selected during monotherapy or with virologic failure in combination with PEG/RBV.[60,61] The barrier to resistance differs between 1a and 1b subtypes for NS5A inhibitors likely because of a functional difference between the subtypes. Variants L31V and Y93H confer phenotypic resistance in vitro in 1a and 1b replicon backgrounds; however, the fold shift in EC_{50} is dramatically different depending on the substitution and position (1a: L31V, 2500-fold; Y93H, 2300-fold. 1b: L31V, 81-fold; Y93H, 145-fold).[62] High fold changes analogous to those seen in the 1a replicon are only achieved with the L31V + Y93H mutant in the 1b replicon (>20,000-fold).[62] IFN-free therapy combining BMS-650032 (PI) and BMS-790052 is successful in subjects with 1b (77%–100% SVR), although failing rapidly with viral resistance in most 1a subjects (36% SVR), lending direct clinical support to the impact of difference in resistance barriers for subtypes on clinical outcomes with IFN-free therapy.[63,64] Cross-resistance is widespread for NS5A inhibitors with GS-5885 and ABT-267 selecting for identical resistant variants in vitro and in clinical trials.[65–67]

IFN-FREE THERAPIES AND RESISTANCE

An increasing number of small IFN-free studies with various combinations of HCV antivirals have been completed. Although the numbers are too small to draw definitive conclusions, several important resistance-related concepts have emerged from these early studies: (1) combinations of two low-resistance barrier compounds (PI + NNI) fail in most subjects[68,69]; (2) the resistance barrier differences between 1a and 1b viruses seem to have a significant impact on PI + NS5A regimens[63]; (3) subjects failing IFN-free regimens do so with multi class-resistant variants present at failure[68,70]; (4) the inclusion of high barrier compounds to regimens, such as NIs, prevents short-term viral breakthrough and resistance[71]; and (5) the addition of RBV to low barrier combinations significantly decreases breakthrough rates.[68]

KEY QUESTIONS AND AREAS FOR FUTURE RESEARCH

Tremendous progress has been made in HCV therapeutics over the last decade, yet knowledge of the clinical impact of HCV resistance remains limited. It is clear the HCV therapeutic field is moving toward IFN-free combination regimens. Several key clinical resistance questions need to be addressed as trials move forward including (1) the impact of baseline resistant variants (and critical thresholds for those variants) on success rates for IFN-free regimens; (2) controlled trials to asses the impact of selected resistant variant during prior therapy on subsequent treatment regimens with cross-resistance to those previously administered; and, contingent on these results, (3) to define clinical cutoffs and the role of resistance testing in clinical practice. As HCV therapy continues to evolve and multiple agents with unique resistance profiles are combined an understanding of HCV resistance will be integral to effective antiviral therapy. Infectious disease physicians and HIV specialists are well suited to dealing with these complexities and are likely to be a major group of treaters for HCV in the future.

REFERENCES

1. Bacon BR, Gordon SC, Lawitz E, et al. Boceprevir for previously treated chronic HCV genotype 1 infection. N Engl J Med 2011;364(13):1207–17.
2. Poordad F, McCone J Jr, Bacon BR, et al. Boceprevir for untreated chronic HCV genotype 1 infection. N Engl J Med 2011;364(13):1195–206.
3. Jacobson IM, McHutchison JG, Dusheiko G, et al. Telaprevir for previously untreated chronic hepatitis C virus infection. N Engl J Med 2011;364(25): 2405–16.
4. Zeuzem S, Andreone P, Pol S, et al. Telaprevir for retreatment of HCV infection. N Engl J Med 2011;364(25):2417–28.
5. Simmonds P. Genetic diversity and evolution of hepatitis C virus: 15 years on. J Gen Virol 2004;85(Pt 11):3173–88.
6. Ogata N, Alter HJ, Miller RH, et al. Nucleotide sequence and mutation rate of the H strain of hepatitis C virus. Proc Natl Acad Sci U S A 1991;88(8):3392–6.
7. Duffy S, Shackelton LA, Holmes EC. Rates of evolutionary change in viruses: patterns and determinants. Nat Rev Genet 2008;9(4):267–76.
8. Neumann AU, Lam NP, Dahari H, et al. Hepatitis C viral dynamics in vivo and the antiviral efficacy of interferon-alpha therapy. Science 1998;282(5386):103–7.
9. Rong L, Dahari H, Ribeiro RM, et al. Rapid emergence of protease inhibitor resistance in hepatitis C virus. Sci Transl Med 2010;2(30):30ra32.
10. Drake JW, Holland JJ. Mutation rates among RNA viruses. Proc Natl Acad Sci U S A 1999;96(24):13910–3.
11. Perelson AS, Neumann AU, Markowitz M, et al. HIV-1 dynamics in vivo: virion clearance rate, infected cell life-span, and viral generation time. Science 1996; 271(5255):1582–6.
12. Lindenbach BD, Rice CM. Unravelling hepatitis C virus replication from genome to function. Nature 2005;436(7053):933–8.
13. Ho DD, Neumann AU, Perelson AS, et al. Rapid turnover of plasma virions and CD4 lymphocytes in HIV-1 infection. Nature 1995;373(6510):123–6.
14. Finzi D, Hermankova M, Pierson T, et al. Identification of a reservoir for HIV-1 in patients on highly active antiretroviral therapy. Science 1997;278(5341): 1295–300.
15. Finzi D, Blankson J, Siliciano JD, et al. Latent infection of CD4 + T cells provides a mechanism for lifelong persistence of HIV-1, even in patients on effective combination therapy. Nat Med 1999;5(5):512–7.
16. Sarrazin C, Kieffer TL, Bartels D, et al. Dynamic hepatitis C virus genotypic and phenotypic changes in patients treated with the protease inhibitor telaprevir. Gastroenterology 2007;132(5):1767–77.
17. Susser S, Welsch C, Wang Y, et al. Characterization of resistance to the protease inhibitor boceprevir in hepatitis C virus-infected patients. Hepatology 2009;50(6): 1709–18.
18. Vertex Pharmaceuticals. Telaprevir 375-mg film-coated tablet for the treatment of genotype 1 chronic hepatitis C antiviral drugs advisory committee briefing document [internet]. 2011. Available at: http://www.fda.gov/downloads/AdvisoryCommittees/ CommitteesMeetingMaterials/Drugs/AntiviralDrugsAdvisoryCommittee/UCM252562. pdf. Accessed April 29, 2011.

19. Merck and Co., Inc. FDA Antiviral Drugs Advisory Committee Meeting Boceprevir Capsules (NDA 202–258) Briefing Document [internet]. 2011. Available at: http://www.google.com/url?sa=t&source=web&cd=1&sqi=2&ved=0CB0QFjAA&url=http%3A%2F%2Fwww.fda.gov%2Fdownloads%2FAdvisoryCommittees%2FCommitteesMeetingMaterials%2FDrugs%2FAntiviralDrugsAdvisoryCommittee%2FUCM252343.pdf&;ei=fhqKTuj8LIS3tgeFo9BJ&usg=AFQjCNFr9KzfbJy3xPQFkBzQkJvR2U4R2w.

20. McHutchison JG, Manns MP, Muir AJ, et al. Telaprevir for previously treated chronic HCV infection. N Engl J Med 2010;362(14):1292–303.

21. Hézode C, Forestier N, Dusheiko G, et al. Telaprevir and peginterferon with or without ribavirin for chronic HCV infection. N Engl J Med 2009;360(18):1839–50.

22. McHutchison JG, Everson GT, Gordon SC, et al. Telaprevir with peginterferon and ribavirin for chronic HCV genotype 1 infection. N Engl J Med 2009;360(18):1827–38.

23. Kwo PY, Lawitz EJ, McCone J, et al. Efficacy of boceprevir, an NS3 protease inhibitor, in combination with peginterferon alfa-2b and ribavirin in treatment-naive patients with genotype 1 hepatitis C infection (SPRINT-1): an open-label, randomised, multicentre phase 2 trial. Lancet 2010;376(9742):705–16.

24. Kieffer TL, Bartels DJ, Sullivan JC, et al. Characterization of resistant variants in treatment-naive and experienced genotype 1 HCV patients in phase 2 trials of telaprevir/Peg-IFN/RBV. Reviews in Antiviral Therapy and Infectious Diseases 2010; 5:6–7.

25. Sullivan JC, De Meyer S, Bartels DJ, et al. Evolution of treatment-emergent resistant variants in telaprevir phase 3 clinical trials. J Hepatol 2011;54(Suppl 1):S4.

26. Barnard R, Zeuzem S, Vierling JM, et al. Analysis of resistance-associated amino acid variants (RAVS) in non-SVR patients enrolled in a retrospective long-term follow-up analysis of boceprevir phase 3 clinical studies. Hepatology 2011; 54(4):440–441A.

27. Sherman KE, Sulkowski MS, Zoulim F, et al. Follow-up of SVR durability and viral resistance in patients with chronic hepatitis C treated with telaprevir-based regimens: interim analysis of the EXTEND study. Hepatology 2011;54(Suppl 4): 485–86S.

28. Zeuzem S, Sulkowski M, Zoulim F, et al. Long-term follow-up of patients with chronic hepatitis c treated with telaprevir in combination with peginterferon alfa-2a and ribavirin: interim analysis of the EXTEND Study. Hepatology 2010; 52(Suppl 4):436A.

29. De Meyer S, Dierynck I, Ghys A, et al. 1202 characterisation of HCV variants in non-SVR patients in the REALIZE study suggests that telaprevir exhibits a consistent resistance profile irrespective of a lead-in. J Hepatol 2011;54(Suppl 1):S475.

30. De Meyer S, Thys K, Dierynck I, et al. 1174 deep sequencing screening for telaprevir-resistant viral variants in previous null responders fails to identify those patients at risk of failing telaprevir plus peginterferon/ribavirin therapy. J Hepatol 2012;56(Suppl 2):S465.

31. Hirsch MS, Günthard HF, Schapiro JM, et al. Antiretroviral drug resistance testing in adult HIV-1 infection: 2008 recommendations of an international AIDS Society-USA Panel. Clin Infect Dis 2008 Jul;47(2):266–85.

32. Little SJ, Holte S, Routy J-P, et al. Antiretroviral-drug resistance among patients recently infected with HIV. N Engl J Med 2002;347(6):385–94.

33. Lorenzi P, Opravil M, Hirschel B, et al. Impact of drug resistance mutations on virologic response to salvage therapy. Swiss HIV Cohort Study. AIDS 1999; 13(2):F17–21.

34. Parkin NT, Lie YS, Hellmann N, et al. Phenotypic changes in drug susceptibility associated with failure of human immunodeficiency virus type 1 (HIV-1) triple combination therapy. J Infect Dis 1999;180(3):865–70.

35. Kuritzkes DR, Lalama CM, Ribaudo HJ, et al. Preexisting resistance to nonnucleoside reverse-transcriptase inhibitors predicts virologic failure of an efavirenz-based regimen in treatment-naive HIV-1-infected subjects. J Infect Dis 2008;197(6): 867–70.

36. Schuurman R, Demeter L, Reichelderfer P, et al. Worldwide evaluation of DNA sequencing approaches for identification of drug resistance mutations in the human immunodeficiency virus type 1 reverse transcriptase. J Clin Microbiol 1999;37(7):2291–6.

37. Fried MW, Buti M, Dore GJ, et al. TMC435 in combination with peginterferon and ribavirin in treatment-naïve HCV genotype 1 patients: final analysis of the pillar phase IIB study. Hepatology 2011;54(Suppl 4):1429A.

38. Sulkowski MS, Asselah T, Ferenci P, et al. Treatment with the second generation HCV protease inhibitor bi201335 results in high and consistent SVR rates: results from silen-c1 in treatment-naïve patients across different baseline factors. Hepatology 2011;54(Suppl 4):473–474A.

39. Lenz O, Verbinnen T, Lin TI, et al. In vitro resistance profile of the hepatitis C virus NS3/4A protease inhibitor TMC435. Antimicrob Agents Chemother 2010;54(5): 1878–87.

40. Lagacé L, White PW, Bousquet C, et al. In vitro resistance profile of the hepatitis C virus NS3 protease inhibitor BI 201335. Antimicrob Agents Chemother 2012; 56(1):569–72.

41. Lin C, Lin K, Luong YP, et al. In vitro resistance studies of hepatitis C virus serine protease inhibitors, VX-950 and BILN 2061: structural analysis indicates different resistance mechanisms. J Biol Chem 2004;279(17):17508–14.

42. Lenz O, de Bruijne J, Vijgen L, et al. 1221 treatment outcome and resistance analysis in HCV genotype 1 patients previously exposed to tmc435 monotherapy and re-treated with tmc435 in combination with pegifnî±-2a/ribavirin. J Hepatol 2011; 54(Suppl 1):S482–3.

43. Kukolj G, Bethell R, Cartier M, et al. 1185 characterization of HCV NS3 variants that emerged during virologic breakthrough and relapse from BI 201335 phase II silen-c2 study in PEGIFN/RBV treatment-experienced patients. J Hepatol 2012;56(Suppl 2):S469.

44. Kukolj G, Legace L, Cartier M, et al. Characterization of HCV NS3 variants that emerged during virologic breakthrough and relapse from BI201335 phase 2 SILEN-C1 study. Hepatology 2011;54(Suppl 4):991A.

45. Pilot-Matias T, Tripathi R, Dekhtyar T, et al. 1229 genotypic and phenotypic characterization of NS3 variants selected in HCV-infected patients treated with ABT-450. J Hepatol 2011;54(Suppl 1):S485–6.

46. Carroll S, McCauley J, Ludmerer S, et al. 39 MK-5172: a novel HCV NS3/4A protease inhibitor with potent activity against known resistance mutants. J Hepatol 2010; 52(Suppl 1):S17.

47. Petry A, Fraser I, O'Mara E, et al. Safety and antiviral activity of MK-5172, a next generation HCV NS3/4A protease inhibitor with a broad hcv genotypic activity spectrum and potent activity against known resistance mutants, in genotype 1 and 3 HCV- infected patients. Hepatology 2011;54(Suppl 4):531A.

48. Howe AY, Cheng H, Thompson I, et al. Molecular mechanism of a thumb domain hepatitis C virus nonnucleoside RNA-dependent RNA polymerase inhibitor. Antimicrob Agents Chemother 2006;50(12):4103–13.

49. Powdrill MH, Bernatchez JA, Götte M. Inhibitors of the hepatitis C virus RNA-dependent RNA polymerase NS5B. Viruses 2010;2(10):2169–95.

50. Margeridon S, Le Pogam S, Liu T, et al. No detection of variants bearing NS5B S282T mericitabine (MCB) resistance mutation in DAA treatment-naive HCV genotype 1 (G1)-infected patients using ultra-deep pyrosequencing (UDPS). Hepatology 2011;54(Suppl 4):532A.

51. Kuntzen T, Timm J, Berical A, et al. Naturally occurring dominant resistance mutations to hepatitis C virus protease and polymerase inhibitors in treatment-naïve patients. Hepatology 2008;48(6):1769–78.

52. Le Pogam S, Seshaadri A, Kosaka A, et al. Existence of hepatitis C virus NS5B variants naturally resistant to non-nucleoside, but not to nucleoside, polymerase inhibitors among untreated patients. J Antimicrob Chemother 2008; 61(6):1205–16.

53. Migliaccio G, Tomassini JE, Carroll SS, et al. Characterization of resistance to non-obligate chain-terminating ribonucleoside analogs that inhibit hepatitis C virus replication in vitro. J Biol Chem 2003;278(49):49164–70.

54. McCown MF, Rajyaguru S, Le Pogam S, et al. The hepatitis C virus replicon presents a higher barrier to resistance to nucleoside analogs than to nonnucleoside polymerase or protease inhibitors. Antimicrob Agents Chemother 2008;52(5): 1604–12.

55. Lam AM, Espiritu C, Bansal S, et al. Genotype and subtype profiling of PSI-7977 as a nucleotide inhibitor of hepatitis C virus [internet]. Antimicrob Agents Chemother 2012. Available at: http://www.ncbi.nlm.nih.gov/pubmed/22430955. Accessed May 1, 2012.

56. Brown NA. Progress towards improving antiviral therapy for hepatitis C with hepatitis C virus polymerase inhibitors. Part I: nucleoside analogues. Expert Opin Investig Drugs 2009;18(6):709–25.

57. Wedemeyer H, Jensen D, Herring R Jr, et al. 1213 efficacy and safety of mericitabine (MCB) in combination with PEG-IFNA-2A/RBV in G1/4 treatment naive HCV patients: final analysis from the PROPEL study. J Hepatol 2012;56(Suppl 2): S481–2.

58. Gane EJ, Stedman CA, Hyland RH, et al. 1113 electron: once daily PSI-7977 Plus RBV in HCV GT1/2/3. J Hepatol 2012;56(Suppl 2):S438–9.

59. Gao M, Nettles RE, Belema M, et al. Chemical genetics strategy identifies an HCV NS5A inhibitor with a potent clinical effect [internet]. Nature 2010. Available at: http://dx.doi.org/10.1038/nature08960. Accessed April 26, 2012.

60. Pol S, Rustgi VK, Martorell C, et al. High rates of SVR24 for BMS-790052, an NS5A replication complex inhibitor, in combination with PegIFN-alfa-2a and ribavirin: phase 2a trial in treatment-naive HCV genotype 1 subjects. Chicago: American Society for Microbiology; 2011.

61. Fridell RA, Wang C, Sun J-H, et al. Genotypic and phenotypic analysis of variants resistant to hepatitis C virus nonstructural protein 5A replication complex inhibitor BMS-790052 in humans: in vitro and in vivo correlations. Hepatology 2011;54(6): 1924–35.

62. Wang C, Huang H, Valera L, et al. Hepatitis C virus RNA elimination and development of resistance in replicon cells treated with BMS-790052. Antimicrob Agents Chemother 2012;56(3):1350–8.

63. Lok AS, Gardiner DF, Lawitz E, et al. Preliminary study of two antiviral agents for hepatitis C genotype 1. N Engl J Med 2012;366(3):216–24.

64. Suzuki F, Ikeda K, Toyota J, et al. 14 dual oral therapy with the NS5A inhibitor DACLATASVIR (BMS-790052) and NS3 protease inhibitor asunaprevir (BMS-650032)

in HCV genotype 1B-infected null responders or ineligible/intolerant to peginterferon/ribavirin. J Hepatol 2012;56(Suppl 2):S7–8.

65. Cheng G, Peng B, Corsa A, et al. 1172 antiviral activity and resistance profile of the novel HCV NS5A inhibitor GS-5885. J Hepatol 2012;56(Suppl 2):S464.

66. Lawitz EJ, Gruener D, Hill JM, et al. A phase 1, randomized, placebo-controlled, 3-day, dose-ranging study of GS-5885, an NS5A inhibitor, in patients with genotype 1 hepatitis C [internet]. J Hepatol 2012. Available at:. http://www.ncbi.nlm.nih.gov/pubmed/22314425. Accessed May 1, 2012.

67. Lawitz E, Marbury T, Campbell A, et al. 1186 safety and antiviral activity of ABT-267, a novel NS5A inhibitor, during 3-day monotherapy: first study in HCV genotype-1 (GT1)-infected treatment-naive subjects. J Hepatol 2012;56(Suppl 2):S469–70.

68. Zeuzem S, Buggisch P, Agarwal K, et al. Dual, triple, and quadruple combination treatment with a protease inhibitor (GS-9256) and a polymerase inhibitor (GS-9190) alone and in combination with ribavirin (RBV) or PegIFN/RBV for up to 28 days in treatment naïve, genotype 1 HCV subjects. Hepatology 2010;52(Suppl 1):A400–1, LB–1.

69. Di Bisceglie AM, Nelson DR, Gane E, et al. 1363 VX-222 with TVR alone or in combination with peginterferon alfa-2a and ribavirin in treatment-naive patients with chronic hepatitis C: zenith study interim results. J Hepatol 2011;54(Suppl 1):S540.

70. McPhee F, Hernandez D, Yu F, et al. 63 characterization of virologic escape in HCV genotype 1 null responders receiving a combination of the NS3 protease inhibitor BMS-650032 and NS5A inhibitor BMS-790052. J Hepatol 2011;54(Suppl 1):S28–9.

71. Gane EJ, Roberts SK, Stedman CA, et al. Oral combination therapy with a nucleoside polymerase inhibitor (RG7128) and danoprevir for chronic hepatitis C genotype 1 infection (INFORM-1): a randomised, double-blind, placebo-controlled, dose-escalation trial [internet]. Lancet 2010. Available at: http://www.ncbi.nlm.nih.gov/pubmed/20951424. Accessed October 21, 2010.

Care of the Cirrhotic Patient

Syed-Mohammed Jafri, MD, Stuart C. Gordon, MD*

KEYWORDS

- Cirrhosis • Antimicrobial therapy • Viral hepatitis • Hepatic decompensation

KEY POINTS

- The clinical manifestations of cirrhosis encompass a broad spectrum of conditions that reflect the consequences of increased portal pressures secondary to fibrosis and diminished hepatic synthetic function.
- Decompensated liver disease traditionally reflects the occurrence of ascites, gastrointestinal hemorrhage, or encephalopathy in the patient with cirrhosis.
- Antimicrobial management of patients with decompensated cirrhosis includes oral prophylaxis for bacterial peritonitis, nonabsorbable oral rifaximin for hepatic encephalopathy, and preemptive intravenous antibiotics in the face of acute gastrointestinal hemorrhage.
- After the development of hepatic decompensation, current hepatitis C antiviral therapy is no longer an option; such therapy is therefore strongly recommended in well-compensated patients with cirrhosis, and successful treatment may lead to improvement of liver function.
- Evaluation for liver transplantation should be initiated after the onset of clinical decompensation (ascites, encephalopathy, bleeding varices); onset of liver cancer; or after the Model for End Stage Liver Disease score exceeds 15.

INTRODUCTION

Cirrhosis occurs when chronic hepatocyte or bile duct injury causes progressive diffuse hepatic fibrosis with the development of regenerative nodules.[1] It is often difficult to label a patient as cirrhotic, because there may only be subtle changes in laboratory parameters. Current imaging modalities in the United States have variable sensitivity for detecting cirrhosis.[2] Physical and laboratory examination may aid in establishing the diagnosis including such signs as palmer erythema, spider angiomata, or splenomegaly, and thrombocytopenia and hypoalbuminemia. However, cirrhosis may occur in the absence of these examinations or laboratory findings, and these parameters are not pathognomonic.

Gastroenterology-Hepatology, Henry Ford Health System, 2799 West Grand Boulevard, Detroit, MI 48202, USA
* Corresponding author.
E-mail address: sgordon3@hfhs.org

Infect Dis Clin N Am 26 (2012) 979–994
http://dx.doi.org/10.1016/j.idc.2012.08.009
id.theclinics.com

Cirrhosis can be presumed in patients with known chronic liver disease and evidence of decompensation including ascites, varices, or hepatic encephalopathy. Liver biopsy remains the gold standard when the clinical, laboratory, and imaging parameters are normal or equivocal. Liver biopsy as an assessment of fibrosis aids in identifying individuals at risk for developing further progressive liver disease. Liver biopsy is most useful in diagnosis with a validated fibrosis staging system, such as Ishak (0–6) or Metavir (0–4) scores.[2] Persons with minimal fibrosis (Metavir 0–1, Ishak 0–2) have low risk for complications and death during 10 to 20 years of follow-up, whereas the presence of bridging fibrosis (Metavir 3, Ishak 4) often predicts imminent progression to cirrhosis (Metavir 4, Ishak 5–6).[3] The risk of cirrhosis development in viral hepatitis C ranges from 5% to 25% during a 25- to 30-year period after virus acquisition.[4–6]

CIRRHOSIS AND ITS COMPLICATIONS
Evaluation of Cirrhosis

The Child-Turcotte-Pugh (CTP) score was initially developed for quantifying the risk of portal caval shunt surgery among alcoholic patients with cirrhosis but has subsequently been validated in patients with other forms of liver disease, including hepatitis C. It assesses the prognosis of chronic liver disease based on degree of abnormalities in bilirubin level, albumin level, the international normalized ratio for prothrombin time (INR), and the degree of hepatic encephalopathy and ascites. More than 30% of patients with CTP scores of 10 or more (class C) can be expected to die within 1 year.[4] In contrast, patients with CTP scores of 7 to 9 (class B) have an 80% chance of surviving 5 years, and those with CTP scores of 5 to 6 (class A) have a 90% chance of surviving more than 5 years without transplant.[7]

The Model for End-Stage Liver Disease (MELD) score was originally developed by investigators at Mayo Clinic to assess prognosis among patients undergoing transjugular intrahepatic portosystemic shunts.[8] The MELD score is computed-based on serum bilirubin (S-bilirubin); serum creatinine (S-creatinine); and INR.[9] The result is a score from 6 to 40, with respective 3-month survival from 90% to 7%.[8] This model assesses prognosis (survival estimates) in patients with cirrhosis, and in the United States is used to prioritize patients for donor allocation.[10,11] The MELD score is useful in predicting short-term survival and the risk of postoperative mortality.[4,5]

DECOMPENSATED CIRRHOSIS

Patients with cirrhosis with Child-Pugh scores less than seven or MELD scores less than 15 who do not have complications caused by hepatic dysfunction are said to have compensated disease.[12] The occurrence of ascites, gastrointestinal hemorrhage, or encephalopathy signals the onset of decompensation in a patient with cirrhosis. Patients with advanced fibrosis (Metavir score of F3 or F4) progress to decompensated liver disease at a rate of approximately 5% per year, progress to hepatocellular carcinoma (HCC) at a rate of 1% to 2% per year, and progress to death at a rate of 3% to 4% per year.[13–16] The 5-year survival of patients with decompensated cirrhosis is 50% compared with 91% in those with compensated cirrhosis.[14]

Many of the physiologic consequences and clinical sequelae of decompensated liver disease are related to alteration in blood flow through the liver. A buildup of fibrotic scar tissue and intrahepatic vasoconstriction in the liver with decrease in nitric oxide can cause reduction of blood flow into the liver. This phenomenon causes blood to back up into the many vessels within the splanchnic circulation that, in turn, results in many of the complications related to decompensation.[17,18]

A patient should be considered for transplantation after the onset of clinical decompensation or after the MELD score exceeds 15.[19] Cirrhotic complications that represent manifestations of decompensation may include the following[20]:

- Ascites
- Hepatic encephalopathy
- Hepatorenal syndrome (resulting from vasoconstriction of the renovascular system leading to renal insufficiency)
- Hepatic hydrothorax (ascitic fluid seeping into the pleural space caused by negative pressure and the porous diaphragm)
- Spontaneous bacterial peritonitis (SBP) caused by dysfunction of the intestinal barrier leading to infection in the low-protein ascitic fluid
- Portopulmonary hypertension caused by thrombotic remodeling of the pulmonary vasculature leading to resistance to flow into the lungs
- Hepatopulmonary syndrome with vasodilatation of the pulmonary arteries leading to shunting and poor oxygenation
- Development of HCC that also, by convention, represents a manifestation of decompensation.

VARICES

A response to reduced blood flow into the liver is the development of collateral vessels. These vessels grow mostly in mucosal junctions with potential resultant varices in the esophagus, stomach, and rectum. Variceal bleed represents the most common lethal complication of cirrhosis. Independent predictors of varices include elevated MELD score; low platelet count (<93,000/mm^3); elevated aspartate aminotransferase (>1.34 times upper limit of normal); and total bilirubin higher than 1 mg/dL.[21] A total of 40% of compensated patients with cirrhosis and 85% of patients with decompensated cirrhosis have varices.[22] Esophageal varices develop in 35% to 80% of patients with cirrhosis, and bleeding occurs in 25% to 40% of those with varices.[23] Patients with advanced fibrosis should be monitored periodically for varices using esophagogastroduodenoscopy (EGD).[24] Those with no varices should have repeat EGD performed at 3 years for well-compensated liver disease and at 1 year for decompensated disease. Patients with small varices may be observed with repeat EGD in 2 years for well-compensated disease and at 1 year for decompensated disease. Patients with medium (<30% of esophageal circumference) or large (>30%) varices who have no red wales (indicating impending bleeding) should receive β-blocker treatment with consideration for endoscopic band ligation.[25,26] Any patient with red wales should be given β-blocker treatment and be treated with esophageal band ligation. Repeat EGD interval for patients undergoing band ligation should be every 2 to 3 weeks until elimination.[25,26]

Patients with bleeding esophageal varices have a 90-day mortality of 30%.[13,23] Acute bleeding episodes are managed with splanchnic vasoconstriction with intravenous octreotide and endoscopic band ligation of varices.[27] Transjugular intrahepatic portosystemic shunt is used as a means of managing bleeding refractory to endoscopic attempts at bleeding control. The procedure is a means of stenting from the portal to the hepatic vein, reducing the resistance created by the cirrhotic liver to relieve pressure in venous collaterals/varices.[28] Patients whose hepatic vein portal gradient is decreased to less than 12 mm Hg have a lower probability of developing recurrent variceal hemorrhage, and a lower risk of developing ascites, SBP, and death. At the same time, such a shunt may increase the probability of hepatic encephalopathy,[29,30] and posttransjugular intrahepatic portosystemic shunts mortality increases with higher MELD scores.

ASCITES AND SBP

Lymphatic drainage is supplemented by blood flow from the peritoneal space into the splanchnic circulation leading to decreased fluid absorption along the peritoneal surface, resulting in ascites.[31] Complications of ascites include hepatorenal syndrome, hepatic hydrothorax, and SBP. Because of the potentially lethal nature of SBP, a diagnostic paracentesis is indicated with any change in a cirrhotic's health status including any hospitalization, a rapid increase in ascites, abdominal discomfort, fever or relative leukocytosis, change in mental status, or gastrointestinal bleeding. Therapeutic taps should be performed only in the case of discomfort or shortness of breath caused by fluid overload and not for cosmetic reasons. A strict low-salt diet (<2000 mg/day) and gentle up-titration of diuretics must be emphasized to prevent excessive reliance on paracenteses.

SBP is diagnosed by examining the ascitic fluid: greater than 250 polymorphonuclear cells/mL, or a positive culture result are indicative of SBP. Paracentesis at the time of hospital admission is important because a high proportion of patients with ascites have SBP at the time of admission, whether or not fever or abdominal discomfort is present, and SBP is associated with marked morbidity and mortality. Paracentesis is very safe regardless of the patient's degree of coagulopathy. There is no need to transfuse fresh frozen plasma or platelets before undergoing the procedure, because these measures do not reduce the low bleeding risk associated with paracentesis.[32]

Cell counts on the fluid should be performed and fluid should be injected directly into bedside culture bottles, because false-negative results occur in 40% to 50% with improper culture technique. Albumin replacement is required if the patient's creatinine level is elevated or if more than 5 L of fluid is removed, because such replacement significantly reduces the morbidity and mortality associated with post-paracentesis circulatory dysfunction.[33]

Literature from 20 years ago suggested that less than half of those in whom SBP develops can be expected to survive 1 year.[34,35] The ascitic fluid polymorphonuclear leukocyte count is more rapidly available than the culture and seems to be accurate in determining the need for empiric antibiotic treatment.[36,37] Delaying antimicrobial treatment until the ascitic fluid culture grows bacteria may prove lethal because of overwhelming infection.

Therapy consists of a 5-day course of intravenous cefotaxime or other cephalosporin.[38–40] For β-lactam allergy, ciprofloxacin can be considered although the incidence of fluoroquinolone resistance is increasing and alterations in therapy may be needed based on ascitic fluid cultures. Recent studies emphasize an increased resistance to cephalosporins and suggest that first-line therapy should include meropenem or piperacillin-tazobactam.[41,42]

The current algorithm for therapy remains initial empiric therapy with cefotaxime or a similar third-generation cephalosporin, with modifications in this initial empiric therapy only if the patient has a prior history of peritonitis with resistant organisms. Similarly, such empiric therapy requires modification pending cultures that demonstrate resistant bacteria or continued evidence of infection (persisting white cell count elevation or persistent bacteria on repeat paracentesis) necessitating the use of broad-spectrum antibiotic regimens. Repeat paracentesis should be performed 72 hours after treatment initiation to check for white blood cell response; absence of response may suggest the presence of an organism with drug resistance or an alternate diagnosis.[40]

Early onset albumin infusions have been shown to reduce mortality through reduction of renal impairment. One study showed a reduction in 60-day mortality from 29% with cefotaxime alone to 10% with cefotaxime plus 1.5 g/kg albumin administered within 6 hours of SBP diagnosis, followed by 1 g/kg on Day 3.[37]

Primary and Secondary SBP Prophylaxis

Antibiotic prophylaxis with ciprofloxacin (750 mg/week) has been shown to prevent SBP in patients with ascites, with one classic study showing a 6-month incidence of SBP of 4% with ciprofloxacin versus 22% with placebo.[43] When first described, the mortality of SBP exceeded 90%; however, with early recognition of the disease and prompt and appropriate antibiotic therapy, mortality has been reduced to around 30%.[41] Alternative antibiotics for prophylaxis are norfloxacin and trimethoprim-sulfamethoxazole. The potential detriment of prophylaxis is a demonstrated increased incidence of fluoroquinolone resistance among patients with cirrhosis patients.[42] The guidelines by the American Association for the Study of Liver Diseases weigh the benefits and risk of antibiotic prophylaxis[44]; there is a strong recommendation for prophylaxis in patients after an occurrence of SBP, yet stopping short of a strong recommendation for primary prophylaxis in patients with cirrhosis with ascites and low ascitic protein (<1 g/dL) who do not have a prior history of infection. Primary prophylaxis studies found no significant difference in the incidence of infections, including SBP, with norfloxacin or ciprofloxacin treatment but significantly lower incidence of gram-negative infections.[45] Intermittent or weekly dosing may select resistant flora more rapidly.[46] Daily dosing of this drug combination is recommended rather than intermittent dosing.[44] Pharmacologic acid suppression with proton pump inhibitors has been demonstrated to increase the incidence of SBP.[47]

ANTIBIOTIC PROPHYLAXIS IN GASTROINTESTINAL BLEED

Antibiotic therapy is an integral part in the management of patients with cirrhosis and gastrointestinal bleeding, because several randomized controlled trials and two meta-analyses have demonstrated a significant reduction in bacterial infections and overall mortality and mortality with this intervention.[48,49] Gastrointestinal hemorrhage is the most frequently overlooked indication for antibiotic prophylaxis.[50] Intravenous ceftriaxone for 7 days or twice-daily oral norfloxacin for 7 days should be given to prevent bacterial infections in patients with cirrhosis and gastrointestinal hemorrhage.[44] Ceftriaxone is the preferred agent because of an increase in quinolone-resistant bacteria in the cirrhotic population. Intravenous ceftriaxone was far superior to oral norfloxacin in the prophylaxis of spontaneous bacteremia or SBP in patients with advanced cirrhosis and hemorrhage.[51]

BACTERIAL INFECTIONS IN CIRRHOSIS

Infection-related mortality ranges from 7% to 40%.[52] Polymorphonuclear leukocyte dysfunction is a crucial multifactorial parameter leading to infection predisposition. Complement deficiency has been attributed to decreased production from a failing liver and to increased consumption because of a constant acute phase response observed in cirrhosis, related to the endotoxin load.[53,54] C3 deficiency is a significant predictor of mortality.[55]

The death rate for bacteremia and sepsis in patients with cirrhosis is higher than noncirrhotics and highest in alcoholic patients with cirrhosis.[56,57] Mortality after septic shock ranges from 55% to 100% and is closely related to the development of renal failure.[58,59] Mortality from respiratory infections is more than 40% with increased Child-Pugh stage representing a risk factor for mortality.[45] Fatality rate for meningitis exceeds 50% with the most common pathogens including *Streptococcus pneumoniae*, *Escherichia coli*, and *Listeria monocytogenes*.[60,61]

The most common bacteria leading to infection in cirrhosis are gram-positives including *Staphylococcus aureus*. These occur most commonly in compensated patients with cirrhosis. Methicillin resistance is progressively more common in the presence of decompensation.[62] *E coli* is the most common cause of infection in Childs C patients, accounting for 20% of urinary infections, with mortality from infections of 48%.[63,64] *Clostridium* infections occur with a higher incidence and a worse prognosis in patients with cirrhosis compared with noncirrhotics (54%–65% vs 19%).[65] *Mycobacterium tuberculosis* has an increased incidence, poorer prognosis, and an increased rate of resistance in patients with cirrhosis, with fatality up to 48%.[66]

In patients with cirrhosis, adrenal insufficiency may develop during sepsis.[67] The 250-μg adrenocorticotropic hormone stimulation test or direct free cortisol measurement or its surrogates may be useful measurements to define adrenal insufficiency in patients with cirrhosis, but further studies are needed to clarify this observation. One smaller study concluded that hydrocortisone (50 mg intravenously every 6 hours) administration in patients with cirrhosis with sepsis was associated with a significantly higher frequency of shock resolution and a higher survival rate.[68]

HEPATIC ENCEPHALOPATHY

The original detection of overt hepatic encephalopathy was diagnosed by the observation of hand asterixis (also known as liver flapping or flapping tremor). It is caused by the shunting of gut-derived neuroactive substances that cross the blood-brain barrier; these substances are mostly nitrogen based and act as inhibitory neurotransmitters. Precipitating factors for hepatic encephalopathy include gastrointestinal bleeding; infection (including SBP); vascular thrombosis; HCC; and narcotics/sedating medications.[69] Traditional but non–Food and Drug Administration approved treatments for hepatic encephalopathy include lactulose or other nonabsorbable sugars, which cause osmotic diarrhea and movement of nitrogen compounds out of the gut; and use of antibiotics, such as neomycin and metronidazole, which change the gut flora.

A recent phase III trial showed that, compared with placebo, the nonabsorbable antibiotic rifaximin administered at 550 mg twice daily was associated with a statistically significant reduction in episodes of breakthrough hepatic encephalopathy in patients in remission from recurrent hepatic encephalopathy (breakthrough episodes occurred in 22.1% of patients taking rifaximin vs 45.9% with placebo; $P < .001$).[70] More than 90% of patients in the trial received concomitant lactulose therapy. Rifaximin is now Food and Drug Administration approved for the treatment of hepatic encephalopathy, and treatment is associated with a significant reduction in frequency of hospitalization for hepatic encephalopathy (13.6% hospitalization rate with rifaximin vs 22.6% with placebo; $P = .01$).

HEPATOCELLULAR CARCINOMA

Although primary hepatic resection has long been considered the treatment of choice for HCC, 5-year tumor-free survival rates are less than 50%.[71] Furthermore, most patients referred for resection are declined, because the tumor is unresectable or because hepatic reserve is considered inadequate.[72] Even in patients with well-compensated cirrhosis, there is an increase in mortality after surgical resection if patients have evidence of portal hypertension or elevated serum bilirubin values.[73] Radiofrequency ablation and percutaneous alcohol injection are effective in tumors smaller than 3 cm but are far less successful for larger tumors.[74,75] In selected patients with otherwise untreatable tumors but relatively well-preserved liver function, chemoembolization has been shown to improve survival; however, these patients have much lower survival rates than those who are candidates for surgical or ablative therapy.[76–78]

Optimal results after transplantation can be achieved in patients with a single lesion less than 5 cm, or no more than three lesions, the largest of which is less than 3 cm in size, and no radiographic evidence of extrahepatic disease.[79] The allocation policy for donor livers in the United States was modified to give such patients enhanced priority for deceased donor organs. Since implementation of this modification, the time on the donor waiting list for patients with HCC has decreased from a mean of 2.3 years to 0.7 months.[80]

Patients with chronic hepatitis B, chronic hepatitis C, and nonalcoholic steatohepatitis are at particularly high risk for HCC.[81] Viral eradication reduces but does not eliminate the risk of HCC. Liver cancer has been reported to occur after viral cure in hepatitis B and C.[82,83] Consequently, the American Association for the Study of Liver Diseases (AASLD) guidelines recommend that patients with cirrhosis should remain on surveillance programs aimed at the early diagnosis of HCC, with imaging of the liver every 6 months.[84]

TREATMENT OF HEPATITIS C IN PATIENTS WITH CIRRHOSIS

Hepatitis C therapy in patients with cirrhosis is approached with the goal of sustained virologic response (SVR) representing eradication of the virus and thereby, in theory, the prevention of liver-related deaths caused by the development of decompensated cirrhosis and HCC.[85–87] Eliminating hepatitis C has been shown to prevent progression to potentially fatal complications by ameliorating portal hypertension, by decreasing the risk for development of HCC, and by leading to fibrosis regression.[87–90] A total of 70% to 88% of patients chronically infected with HCV do not undergo treatment because of poor health access, medical contraindications including psychiatric or cardiac disease, and patient preference.[91–95]

Guidelines strongly recommend antiviral treatment for patients with more advanced fibrosis and cirrhosis given their increased risk of liver-related complications.[96,97] Patients with compensated HCV related liver disease should be treated provided serum albumin is greater than 3.4 g/dL; bilirubin less than 1.5 mg/dL; INR less than 1.5; platelet count greater than 75,000/mm^3; hemoglobin (Hb) greater than 12/13 g/dL (males 12 g/dL, females 13 g/dL); and S-creatinine less than 1.5 mg/dL. However, the SVR is generally lower and adverse events necessitating dose reductions are higher in patients with cirrhosis.[98,99]

Ideal hepatitis C cirrhosis candidates for therapy remain Child-Pugh class A patients whose virologic response rate is reasonably high and in whom the risk of side effects is almost identical to that of control subjects.[100] Antiviral therapy is currently not indicated in Child-Pugh class C patients (or MELD >18) because of the high risk of sepsis during treatment and a low SVR rate. In Child-Pugh class B patients, treatment should be discussed on a case-by-case basis according to baseline factors for a potential response: genotype non-1, low viral load, good-response IL28B genotype, treatment naive, or patients who have relapsed from previous antiviral therapy. Antiviral therapy can be discontinued after 4 or 12 weeks if there is no virologic response.[101]

The safety of peginterferon therapy is a major concern in patients with advanced or decompensated cirrhosis. The incidence of bacterial infection (either SBP or spontaneous bacteremia) in people with cirrhosis is higher in treated patients (25%) than in control subjects (6%) (P = .01).[102] The development of sepsis is not necessarily related to neutropenia. Splenomegaly caused by portal hypertension increases the risk for cytopenia, especially anemia (35%), neutropenia (38%), and thrombocytopenia (24%).[103,104] The reported rates of neutropenia, thrombocytopenia, anemia, and episodes of infection or liver decompensation during interferon based therapy are 50% to 60%, 30% to 50%, 30% to 60%, 4% to 13%, and 11% to 20%, respectively.[105–107]

The reported rate of clinical decompensation in compensated patients with cirrhosis enrolled in randomized controlled trials is negligible (0%–3%; median, 1.5%)[108] likely reflecting a careful selection of patients with the exclusion of those with advanced liver disease who were at heightened risk of decompensation (rate, 14%).[109] In a prospective controlled trial in patients with decompensated cirrhosis, peginterferon and ribavirin were administered in 66 patients for 24 weeks after patients achieved clinical recompensation (Child-Pugh <9; MELD <15) compared with 63 patients refusing therapy.[110] SVR was 44% for genotypes 2/3 and 7% for genotypes 1/4. Treatment was associated with a risk of infections (odds ratio = 2.43) and death related to infections (odds ratio = 1.97). There was a lower rate of decompensation and reduced mortality in responders.

Guidelines now recommend the addition of a protease inhibitor (boceprevir or telaprevir) to peginterferon and ribavirin for treatment of hepatitis C, genotype 1.[111] These triple therapy regimens yield higher SVR rates, although the SVR rates in patients with cirrhosis are still uncertain because of low numbers of patients with established cirrhosis in the published studies.[112–117] In phase 3 trials, in treatment of naive patients with cirrhosis (6% of study patients), SVR was obtained in 62% of patients treated with telaprevir (12 weeks) compared with 33% with the standard treatment regimen.[116] SVR was achieved in 52% of patients with Metavir score 3 or 4 (around 10% of study patients) treated with boceprevir (44 weeks) compared with 38% with the standard regimen.[115]

In patients with cirrhosis who were previously treated with PEG/ribavirin therapy, SVR was achieved (1) in 84% of those who had relapsed and were now treated with telaprevir compared with 13% who were retreated with the PEG/ribavirin regimen; (2) in 34% of those with a previous partial response treated with telaprevir compared with 20% with PEG/ribavirin; and (3) in 14% of those with a previous nonresponse (reduction of less than 2 $\log_{10}$ in hepatitis C virus [HCV] RNA after 12 weeks) treated with telaprevir compared with 10% with PEG/ribavirin.[118] Interestingly, SVR rates among patients with cirrhosis with prior relapse were comparable with those without cirrhosis in the triple therapy arm, in contrast to the null responders with cirrhosis who did extremely poorly.

In previously treated patients with prior partial response and a baseline Metavir fibrosis score of 3 or 4, SVR was achieved in 83% of those who had relapsed and were treated with boceprevir (44 weeks) compared with 20% with PEG/ribavirin and in 46% of those with a previous nonresponse treated with boceprevir (44 weeks) compared with 0% with PEG/ribavirin.[119] There is no published experience on the efficacy and safety of telaprevir or boceprevir in patients with decompensated cirrhosis and this use is not recommended.[107]

A recent French study investigating telaprevir and boceprevir use in compensated patients with cirrhosis with a history of prior treatment failure supported the increased risk of morbidity and mortality of this therapy in patients with cirrhosis, with serious adverse events (31%–50%) far higher than previously reported.[120] Additional details regarding this unique and important cohort of patients are awaited.

LIVER TRANSPLANTATION

Liver transplantation remains the definitive management for decompensated liver disease.[121] Decompensated cirrhosis caused by HCV accounted for 30% to 50% of the transplants performed in the United States and Europe.[122,123] Survival rates 1, 5, and 10 years after liver transplantation in the United States are 88.9%, 73.6%, and 60.4%, respectively.[124] Patients with a MELD score of 15 or more and a CTP score of 7 or more can be expected to achieve improved survival with liver transplantation.[4,5]

Recurrence of HCV after liver transplantation is universal and follows a more aggressive course than pretransplant HCV infection.[4,5] Most patients with hepatitis C develop recurrent liver injury.[125,126] Postoperative survival in early studies seemed to approximate that of patients transplanted for other conditions.[127] Significant strides have been made in posttransplant therapy for hepatitis B including improved oral antiviral suppression aiding graft survival. With newer direct-acting antivirals for hepatitis C, the hope is that likewise further improvement in graft survival may be achieved in patients with hepatitis C, both pretransplant and posttransplant. Although many patients do well with minimal liver damage despite persistently high levels of circulating virus, presently about 10% of patients develop rapidly progressive fibrosis and cirrhosis within the first few years after transplantation.[128–130]

SUMMARY

The hallmark of liver failure in the patient with cirrhosis, defined as hepatic decompensation, clinically represents the development of ascites, encephalopathy, gastrointestinal bleeding, and carcinoma. Literature from the past decade demonstrates that the infectious disease specialist is instrumental in the appropriate management of the patient with advanced liver disease. Antimicrobial treatment of the patient with cirrhosis in 2012 that reduces complications and improves survival now encompasses SBP diagnosis and prophylaxis, encephalopathy treatment and prophylaxis, and prevention of infection during gastrointestinal bleeding. Careful management of hepatitis antiviral therapy is of paramount importance in patients with cirrhosis patients. Liver transplantation, with subsequent immunosuppression, represents definitive management when medical therapy fails to achieve hepatic compensation.

Principles of management for cirrhotic patients	
Principles of Management for Patients with Cirrhosis	**Refs.**
Antibiotic prophylaxis against bacteria during gastrointestinal hemorrhage	44
Antibiotic prophylaxis after any episode of SBP	44
Albumin infusion at diagnosis and 3 days after SBP	37
Rifaximin 550 mg twice daily with lactulose titration for hepatic encephalopathy	41
Abdominal imaging every 6 months in all patients with cirrhosis	82–84
Hepatitis C therapy in advanced fibrosis with no contraindication	96
Consideration for liver transplant listing for MELD >15 or decompensation	4
Band ligation or β blockade for large varices or varices with red wales	26

REFERENCES

1. Heidelbaugh JJ, Bruderly M. Cirrhosis and chronic liver failure. Part I. Diagnosis and evaluation. Am Fam Physician 2006;74:756–62.
2. Ishak K, Baptista A, Bianchi L, et al. Histological grading and staging of chronic hepatitis. J Hepatol 1995;22:696–9.
3. Vigano M, Lampertico P, Rumi MG, et al. Natural history and clinical impact of cryoglobulins in chronic hepatitis C: 10-year prospective study of 343 patients. Gastroenterology 2007;133:835–42.
4. Freeman RB, Wiesner RH, Edwards E, et al. Results of the first year of the new liver allocation plan. Liver Transpl 2004;10:7–15.
5. Wiesner R, Edwards E, Freeman R, et al. Model for end-stage liver disease (MELD) and allocation of donor livers. Gastroenterology 2003;124:91–6.
6. Shetty K, Rybicki L, Carey WD. The Child-Pugh classification as a prognostic indicator for survival in primary sclerosing cholangitis. Hepatology 1997;25:1049–53.
7. Pugh RN, Murray-Lyon IM, Dawson JL, et al. Transection of the oesophagus for bleeding oesophageal varices. Br J Surg 1973;60:646–8.
8. Malinchoc M, Kamath PS, Gordon FD, et al. A model to predict poor survival in patients undergoing transjugular intrahepatic portosystemic shunts. Hepatology 2000;31:864–71.
9. Kamath PS, Kim WR, Advanced Liver Disease Study Group. The model for end-stage liver disease (MELD). Hepatology 2007;45:797–805.
10. Available at: http://www.mayoclinic.org/meld/mayomodel6.html. Accessed April 6, 2012.
11. Kamath PS, Wiesner RH, Malinchoc M, et al. A model to predict survival in patients with end-stage liver disease. Hepatology 2001;33:464–70.
12. Shah VH, Kamath PS. Portal hypertension and gastrointestinal bleeding. In: Feldman M, Friedman LS, Brandt LJ, editors. Sleisenger and Fordtran's gastrointestinal and liver disease. 8th edition. Philadelphia: Saunders; 2006. p. 1899–934.
13. Sherman KE. Advanced liver disease: what every hepatitis C virus treater should know. Top Antivir Med 2011;19(3):121–5.
14. Fattovich G, Giustina G, Degos F, et al. Morbidity and mortality in compensated cirrhosis type C: a retrospective follow-up study of 384 patients. Gastroenterology 1997;112:463–72.
15. Serfaty L, Aumaître H, Chazouillères O, et al. Determinants of outcome of compensated hepatitis C virus-related cirrhosis. Hepatology 1998;27:1435–40.
16. Hu KQ, Tong MJ. The long-term outcomes of patients with compensated hepatitis C virus-related cirrhosis and history of parenteral exposure in the United States. Hepatology 1999;29:1311–6.
17. Bhathal PS, Grossman HJ. Reduction of the increased portal vascular resistance of the isolated perfused cirrhotic rat liver by vasodilators. J Hepatol 1985;1:325–37.
18. Gupta TK, Chung MK, Toruner M, et al. Endothelial dysfunction in the intrahepatic microcirculation of the cirrhotic rat. Hepatology 1998;28:926–31.
19. Ghany MG, Strader DB, Thomas DL, et al. AASLD practice guidelines: diagnosis, management and treatment of hepatitis C: an update. Hepatology 2009;49:1335–74.

20. Machicao VI, Fallon MB. Hepatopulmonary syndrome. Semin Respir Crit Care Med 2012;33(1):11–6.
21. Tafarel JR, Tolentino LH, Correa LM, et al. Prediction of esophageal varices in hepatic cirrhosis by noninvasive markers. Eur J Gastroenterol Hepatol 2011; 23(9):754–8.
22. Pagliaro L, D'Amico G, Pasta L, et al. Portal hypertension in cirrhosis: natural history. In: Bosch J, Groszmann RJ, editors. Portal hypertension. pathophysiology and treatment. Oxford (United Kingdom): Blackwell Scientific; 1994. p. 72–92.
23. The North Italian Endoscopic Club for the Study and Treatment of Esophageal Varices. Prediction of the first variceal hemorrhage in patients with cirrhosis of the liver and esophageal varices. A prospective multicenter study. N Engl J Med 1988;319:983–9.
24. de Franchis R. Evolving Consensus in Portal Hypertension Report of the Baveno IV Consensus Workshop on methodology of diagnosis and therapy in portal hypertension. J Hepatol 2005;43:167–76.
25. Grace ND, Groszmann RJ, Garcia-Tsao G, et al. Portal hypertension and variceal bleeding: an AASLD single topic symposium. Hepatology 1998;28: 868–80.
26. D'Amico G, Garcia-Tsao G, Cales P, et al. Diagnosis of portal hypertension: how and when. In: de Franchis R, editor. Portal hypertension III. Proceedings of the third baveno international consensus workshop on definitions, methodology and therapeutic strategies. Oxford (United Kingdom): Blackwell Science; 2001. p. 36–64.
27. Sempere L, Palazón JM, Sánchez-Payá J, et al. Assessing the short- and long-term prognosis of patients with cirrhosis and acute variceal bleeding. Rev Esp Enferm Dig 2009;101(4):236–48.
28. Boyer TD, Haskal ZJ. The role of transjugular intrahepatic portosystemic shunt in the management of portal hypertension. Hepatology 2005;41:386–400.
29. Abraldes JG, Tarantino I, Turnes J, et al. Hemodynamic response to pharmacological treatment of portal hypertension and long-term prognosis of cirrhosis. Hepatology 2003;37:902–8.
30. García-Pagán JC, Caca K, Bureau C, et al, Early TIPS (Transjugular Intrahepatic Portosystemic Shunt) Cooperative Study Group. Early use of TIPS in patients with cirrhosis and variceal bleeding. N Engl J Med 2010;362:2370–9.
31. Arroyo V, Colmenero J. Ascites and hepatorenal syndrome in cirrhosis: pathophysiological basis of therapy and current management. J Hepatol 2003;38: S69–89.
32. Runyon BA. Paracentesis of ascitic fluid: a safe procedure. Arch Intern Med 1986;146:2259–61.
33. Bernardi M, Caraceni P, Navickis RJ. Albumin infusion in patients undergoing large-volume paracentesis: a meta-analysis of randomized trials. Hepatology 2012;55:1172–81.
34. Andreu M, Sola R, Sitges SA, et al. Risk factors for spontaneous bacterial peritonitis in cirrhotic patients with ascites. Gastroenterology 1993;104:1133–8.
35. Gines A, Escorsell A, Gines P, et al. Incidence, predictive factors, and prognosis of the hepatorenal syndrome in cirrhosis with ascites. Gastroenterology 1993; 105:229–36.
36. Felisart J, Rimola A, Arroyo V, et al. Randomized comparative study of efficacy and nephrotoxicity of ampicillin plus tobramycin versus cefotaxime in cirrhotics with severe infections. Hepatology 1985;5:457–62.

37. Sort P, Navasa M, Arroyo V, et al. Effect of intravenous albumin on renal impairment and mortality in patients with cirrhosis and spontaneous bacterial peritonitis. N Engl J Med 1999;341:403–9.
38. Fernandez J, Acevedo J, Castro M. Prevalence and risk factors of infections by multiresistant bacteria in cirrhosis: a prospective study. Hepatology 2012;55: 1551–61.
39. Hoefs JC, Canawati HN, Sapico FL, et al. Spontaneous bacterial peritonitis. Hepatology 1982;2:399–407.
40. Runyon BA. Ascites and spontaneous bacterial peritonitis. In: Feldman M, Friedman LS, Brandt LJ, editors. Sleisenger and Fortran's gastrointestinal and liver disease. 8th edition. Philadelphia: Saunders; 2006. p. 1935–64.
41. Garcia-Tsao G. Spontaneous bacterial peritonitis: a historical perspective. J Hepatol 2004;41:522–7.
42. Ariza X, Castellote J, Lora-Tamayo J. Risk factors for resistance to ceftriaxone and its impact on mortality in community, healthcare and nosocomial spontaneous bacterial peritonitis. J Hepatol 2012;56(4):825–32.
43. Rolachon A, Cordier L, Bacq Y, et al. Ciprofloxacin and long-term prevention of spontaneous bacterial peritonitis: results of a prospective controlled trial. Hepatology 1995;22:1171–4.
44. Runyon BA, AASLD Practice Guidelines Committee. Management of adult patients with ascites due to cirrhosis: an update. Hepatology 2009;49:2087–107.
45. Segarra-Newnham M, Henneman A. Antibiotic prophylaxis for prevention of spontaneous bacterial peritonitis in patients without gastrointestinal bleeding. Ann Pharmacother 2010;44:1946–54.
46. Terg R, Llano K, Cobas S, et al. Effect of oral ciprofloxacin on aerobic gram-negative flora of cirrhotic patients: results of short and long term administration with variable dose. Hepatology 1996;24:455A.
47. Goel GA, Deshpande A, Lopez R, et al. Increased rate of spontaneous bacterial peritonitis among cirrhotic patients receiving pharmacologic acid suppression. Clin Gastroenterol Hepatol 2012;10:422–7.
48. Chavez-Tapia NC, Barrientos-Gutierrez T, Tellez-Avila F, et al. Meta-analysis: antibiotic prophylaxis for cirrhotic patients with upper gastrointestinal bleeding. An updated Cochrane review. Aliment Pharmacol Ther 2011;34:509–18.
49. Soares-Weiser K, Brezis M, Tur-Kaspa R, et al. Antibiotic prophylaxis for cirrhotic patients with gastrointestinal bleeding. Cochrane Database Syst Rev 2002;(2):CD002907.
50. Ngamruengphong S, Nugent K, Rakvit A, et al. Potential preventability of spontaneous bacterial peritonitis. Dig Dis Sci 2011;56(9):2728–34.
51. Fernández J, Ruiz del Arbol L, Gómez C, et al. Norfloxacin vs ceftriaxone in the prophylaxis of infections in patients with advanced cirrhosis and hemorrhage. Gastroenterology 2006;131(4):1049–56.
52. Christou L, Pappas G, Falagas ME. Bacterial infection-related morbidity and mortality in cirrhosis. Am J Gastroenterol 2007;102:1510–7.
53. Rimola A, Soto R, Bory F, et al. Reticuloendothelial system phagocytic activity in cirrhosis and its relation to bacterial infections and prognosis. Hepatology 1984; 4:53–8.
54. Akalin HE, Laleli Y, Telatar H. Serum bactericidal and opsonic activities in patients with non-alcoholic cirrhosis. Q J Med 1985;56:431–7.
55. Homann C, Varming K, Hogasen K, et al. Acquired C3 deficiency in patients with alcoholic cirrhosis predisposes to infection and increased mortality. Gut 1997; 40:544–9.

56. Linderoth G, Jepsen P, Schonheyder HC, et al. Short-term prognosis of community-acquired bacteremia in patients with liver cirrhosis or alcoholism: a population-based cohort study. Alcohol Clin Exp Res 2006;30:636–41.

57. Olson JC, Wendon JA, Kramer DJ, et al. Intensive care of the patient with cirrhosis. Hepatology 2011;54:1864–72.

58. Terra C, Guevara M, Torre A, et al. Renal failure in patients with cirrhosis and sepsis unrelated to spontaneous bacterial peritonitis: value of MELD score. Gastroenterology 2005;129:1944–53.

59. Caly WR, Strauss E. A prospective study of bacterial infections in patients with cirrhosis. J Hepatol 1993;18:353–8.

60. Molle I, Thulstrup AM, Svendsen N, et al. Risk and case fatality rate of meningitis in patients with liver cirrhosis. Scand J Infect Dis 2000;32:407–10.

61. Pauwels A, Pines E, Abboura M, et al. Bacterial meningitis in cirrhosis: review of 16 cases. J Hepatol 1997;27:830–4.

62. Campillo B, Richardet JP, Kheo T, et al. Nosocomial spontaneous bacterial peritonitis and bacteremia in cirrhotic patients: impact of isolate type on prognosis and characteristics of infection. Clin Infect Dis 2002;35:1–10.

63. Amdal T, Skinhoj P, Friis H. Bacteremia in patients suffering from cirrhosis. Infection 1986;14:68–70.

64. Frenandez J, Navasa M, Gomez J, et al. Bacterial infections in cirrhosis: epidemiological changes with invasive procedures and norfloxacin prophylaxis. Hepatology 2002;35:140–8.

65. Chen YM, Lee HC, Chang CM, et al. Clostridium bacteremia: emphasis on the poor prognosis in cirrhotic patients. J Microbiol Immunol Infect 2001;34:113–8.

66. Arevalo M, Solera J, Cebrian D, et al. Risk factors associated with drug-resistant *Mycobacterium tuberculosis* in Castillala-Mancha. Eur Respir J 1996;9:274–8.

67. Fede G, Spadaro L, Tomaselli T, et al. Adrenocortical dysfunction in liver disease: a systematic review. Hepatology 2012;55(4):1282–91.

68. Fernández J, Escorsell A, Zabalza M, et al. Adrenal insufficiency in patients with cirrhosis and septic shock: effect of treatment with hydrocortisone on survival. Hepatology 2006;44:1288–95.

69. Sharma P, Singh S, Sharma BC. Propofol sedation during endoscopy in patients with cirrhosis, and utility of psychometric tests and critical flicker frequency in assessment of recovery from sedation. Endoscopy 2011;43(5):400–5.

70. Bass NM, Mullen KD, Sanyal A, et al. Rifaximin treatment in hepatic encephalopathy. N Engl J Med 2010;362:1071–81.

71. Cha CH, Ruo L, Fong Y, et al. Resection of hepatocellular carcinoma in patients otherwise eligible for transplantation. Ann Surg 2003;238:315–21.

72. Bruix J, Sherman M, Llovet JM, et al. Clinical management of hepatocellular carcinoma. Conclusions of the Barcelona-2000 EASL conference. European Association for the Study of the Liver. J Hepatol 2001;35:421–30.

73. Llovet JM, Fuster J, Bruix J. Intention-to-treat analysis of surgical treatment for early hepatocellular carcinoma: resection versus transplantation. Hepatology 1999;30:1434–40.

74. Castells A, Bruix J, Bru C, et al. Treatment of small hepatocellular carcinoma in cirrhotic patients: a cohort study comparing surgical resection and percutaneous ethanol injection. Hepatology 1993;18:1121–6.

75. Curley SA, Izzo F, Ellis LM, et al. Radiofrequency ablation of hepatocellular cancer in 110 patients with cirrhosis. Ann Surg 2000;232:381–91.

76. Llovet JM, Real MI, Montana X, et al. Arterial embolisation or chemoembolisation versus symptomatic treatment in patients with unresectable hepatocellular carcinoma: a randomised controlled trial. Lancet 2002;359:1734–9.

77. Lo CM, Ngan H, Tso WK, et al. Randomized controlled trial of transarterial lipiodol chemoembolization for unresectable hepatocellular carcinoma. Hepatology 2002;35:1164–71.

78. Llovet JM, Bruix J. Systematic review of randomized trials for unresectable hepatocellular carcinoma: chemoembolization improves survival. Hepatology 2003;37:429–42.

79. Mazzaferro V, Regalia E, Doci R, et al. Liver transplantation for the treatment of small hepatocellular carcinomas in patients with cirrhosis. N Engl J Med 1996; 334:693–9.

80. Sharma P, Balan V, Hernandez JL, et al. Liver transplantation for hepatocellular carcinoma: the MELD impact. Liver Transpl 2004;10:36–41.

81. Llovet JM, Bru C, Bruix J. Prognosis of hepatocellular carcinoma: the BCLC staging classification. Semin Liver Dis 1999;19:329–38.

82. Cardoso AC, Moucari R, Figueiredo-Mendes C, et al. Impact of peginterferon and ribavirin therapy on hepatocellular carcinoma: incidence and survival in hepatitis C patients with advanced fibrosis. J Hepatol 2010;52:652–7.

83. Simonetti J, Bulkow L, McMahon BJ, et al. Clearance of hepatitis B surface antigen and risk of hepatocellular carcinoma in a cohort chronically infected with hepatitis B virus. Hepatology 2010;51:1531–7.

84. Bruix J, Sherman M, for the Practical Guidelines Committee. American Association for the Study of Liver Diseases. Management of hepatocellular carcinoma. Available at: https://www.aasld.org/practiceguidelines/Pages/default.aspx. Accessed April 16, 2012.

85. Shindo M, Hamada K, Oda Y, et al. Long-term follow-up study of sustained biochemical responders with interferon therapy. Hepatology 2001;33:1299–302.

86. Yoshida H, Arakawa Y, Sata M, et al. Interferon therapy prolonged life expectancy among chronic hepatitis C patients. Gastroenterology 2002;123: 483–91.

87. Bruno S, Stroffolini T, Colombo M, et al, Italian Association of the Study of the Liver Disease (AISF). Sustained virological response to interferon-alpha is associated with improved outcome in HCV-related cirrhosis: a retrospective study. Hepatology 2007;45:579–87.

88. Rincon D, Ripoll C, Lo Iacono O, et al. Antiviral therapy decreases hepaticvenous pressure gradient in patients with chronic hepatitis C and advanced fibrosis. Am J Gastroenterol 2006;101:2269–74.

89. Miyake Y, Takaki A, Iwasaki Y, et al. Meta-analysis: interferon-alpha prevents the recurrence after curative treatment of hepatitis C virus-related hepatocellular carcinoma. J Viral Hepat 2010;17:287–92.

90. Heathcote EJ, Shiffman ML, Cooksley WG, et al. Peginterferon alfa-2a in patients with chronic hepatitis C and cirrhosis. N Engl J Med 2000;343:1673–80.

91. Morrill JA, Shrestha M, Grant RW. Barriers to the treatment of hepatitis C. Patient, provider, and system factors. J Gen Intern Med 2005;20:754–8.

92. Butt AA, Wagener M, Shakil AO, et al. Reasons for non-treatment of hepatitis C in veterans in care. J Viral Hepat 2005;12:81–5.

93. Falck-Ytter Y, Kale H, Mullen KD, et al. Surprisingly small effect of antiviral treatment in patients with hepatitis C. Ann Intern Med 2002;136:288–92.

94. Shehab TM, Orrego M, Chunduri R, et al. Identification and management of hepatitis C patients in primary care clinics. Am J Gastroenterol 2003;98:639–44.

95. Butt AA, Justice AC, Skanderson M, et al. Rate and predictors of treatment prescription for hepatitis C. Gut 2007;56:385–9.
96. National Institutes of Health. National Institutes of Health Consensus development conference statement: management of hepatitis C: June 10–12, 2002. Hepatology 2002;36:S3–20.
97. Fried MW. Side effects of therapy of hepatitis C and their management. Hepatology 2002;36:S237–44.
98. Dienstag JL, McHutchison JG. American Gastroenterological Association technical review on the management of hepatitis C. Gastroenterology 2006;130:231–64.
99. Clark BT, Garcia-Tsao G, Fraenkel L. Patterns and predictors of treatment initiation and completion in patients with chronic hepatitis C virus infection. Patient Prefer Adherence 2012;6:285–95.
100. Forns X, Bruix J. Treating hepatitis C in patients with cirrhosis: the effort is worth it. J Hepatol 2010;52:624–6.
101. Somasundaram A, Venkataraman J. Antiviral treatment for cirrhosis due to hepatitis C: a review. Singapore Med J 2012;53(4):231–5.
102. Carrion JA, Martinez-Bauer E, Crespo G, et al. Antiviral therapy increases the risk of bacterial infections in HCV-infected cirrhotic patients awaiting liver transplantation: a retrospective study. J Hepatol 2009;50:719–28.
103. Di Marco V, Almasio PL, Ferraro D, et al. Peg-interferon alone or combined with ribavirin in HCV cirrhosis with portal hypertension: a randomized controlled trial. J Hepatol 2007;47:484–91.
104. Roffi L, Colloredo G, Pioltelli P, et al, for the Gruppo Epatologico Lombardo. Pegylated interferon alpha2b plus ribavirin: an efficacious and well-tolerated treatment regimen for patients with hepatitis C virus related histologically proven cirrhosis. Antivir Ther 2008;13:663–73.
105. Forns X, Garcia-Retortillo M, Serrano T, et al. Antiviral therapy of patients with decompensated cirrhosis to prevent recurrence of hepatitis C after liver transplantation. J Hepatol 2003;39:389–96.
106. Everson GT, Trotter J, Forman L, et al. Treatment of advanced hepatitis C with a low accelerating dosage regimen of antiviral therapy. Hepatology 2005;42:255–62.
107. Roche B, Samuel D. Hepatitis C virus treatment pre- and post-liver transplantation. Liver Int 2012;32(Suppl 1):120–8.
108. Giannini EG, Basso M, Savarino V, et al. Predictive value of ontreatment response during full-dose antiviral therapy of patients with hepatitis C virus cirrhosis and portal hypertension. J Intern Med 2009;266:537–46.
109. Vezali E, Aghemo A, Colombo M. A review of the treatment of chronic hepatitis C virus infection in cirrhosis. Clin Ther 2010;32:2117–38.
110. Iacobellis A, Siciliano M, Perri F, et al. Peginterferon alfa-2b and ribavirin in patients with hepatitis C virus and decompensated cirrhosis: a controlled study. J Hepatol 2007;46:206–12.
111. Ghany MG, Nelson DR, Strader DB, et al, American Association for Study of Liver Diseases. An update on treatment of genotype 1 chronic hepatitis C virus infection: 2011 practice guideline by the American Association for the Study of Liver Diseases. Hepatology 2011;54:1433–44.
112. McHutchison JG, Everson GT, Gordon SC, et al, PROVE1 Study Team. Telaprevir with peginterferon and ribavirin for chronic HCV genotype 1 infection. N Engl J Med 2009;360:1827–38.
113. Hézode C, Forestier N, Dusheiko G, et al, PROVE2 Study Team. Telaprevir and peginterferon with or without ribavirin for chronic HCV infection. N Engl J Med 2009;360:1839–50.

114. Kwo PY, Lawitz EJ, McCone J, et al, SPRINT-1 investigators. Efficacy of boce-previr, an NS3 protease inhibitor, in combination with peginterferon alfa-2b and ribavirin in treatment-naive patients with genotype 1 hepatitis C infection (SPRINT-1): an open-label, randomised, multicentre phase 2 trial. Lancet 2010;376:705–16.

115. Poordad F, McCone J Jr, Bacon BR, et al. Boceprevir for untreated chronic HCV genotype 1 infection. N Engl J Med 2011;364:1195–206.

116. Jacobson IM, McHutchison JG, Dusheiko G, et al, ADVANCE Study Team. Telaprevir for previously untreated chronic hepatitis C virus infection. N Engl J Med 2011;364:2405–16.

117. Sherman KE, Flamm SL, Afdhal NH, et al, ILLUMINATE Study Team. Response-guided telaprevir combination treatment for hepatitis C virus infection. N Engl J Med 2011;365:1014–24.

118. Zeuzem S, Andreone P, Pol S, et al. Telaprevir for retreatment of HCV infection. N Engl J Med 2011;364:2417–28.

119. Bacon BR, Gordon SC, Lawitz E, et al. Boceprevir for previously treated chronic HCV genotype 1 infection. N Engl J Med 2011;364:1207–17.

120. Hezode C, Dorival C, Zoulim F, et al. Telaprevir French cohort authorization for temporary use in genotype 1 hepatitis. J Hepatol 2012;56:S4.

121. Collins BH, Pirsch JD, Becker YT, et al. Long-term results of liver transplantation in patients 60 years of age and older. Transplantation 2000;70:780–3.

122. Berenguer M. Hepatitis C after liver transplantation: risk factors, outcomes, and treatment. Curr Opin Organ Transplant 2005;10:81–9.

123. Samuel D, Forns X, Berenguer M, et al. Report of the monothematic EASL conference on liver transplantation for viral hepatitis (Paris, France, January 12-14, 2006). J Hepatol 2006;45:127–43.

124. Available at: http://www.srtr.org/annual_reports/2010/914a_can-abo_li.htm. Accessed April 14, 2012.

125. Gane EJ, Portman BC, Naoumov NV, et al. Long-term outcome of hepatitis C infection after liver transplantation. N Engl J Med 1996;334:815–20.

126. Shuhart MC, Bronner MP, Gretch DR, et al. Histological and clinical outcome after liver transplantation for hepatitis C. Hepatology 1997;26:1646–52.

127. Boker KH, Dalley G, Bahr M, et al. Long-term outcome of hepatitis C virus infection after liver transplantation. Hepatology 1997;25:203–10.

128. Berenguer M. Natural history of recurrent hepatitis C. Liver Transpl 2002;8:S14–8.

129. Testa G, Crippin JS, Netto GJ, et al. Liver transplantation for hepatitis C: recurrence and disease progression in 300 patients. Liver Transpl 2000;6:553–61.

130. Murray KF, Carithers RL. AASLD Practice Guidelines: evaluation of the patient for liver transplantation. Hepatology 2005;41:1407–32.

Diagnosis and Treatment of Acute Hepatitis C Virus Infection

Christoph Boesecke, MD[a], Heiner Wedemeyer, MD[b],
Jürgen Kurt Rockstroh, MD[a],*

KEYWORDS

- Hepatitis C virus • HIV • Injection drug use • Monoinfection • Coinfection
- Acute hepatitis C

KEY POINTS

- The first 6 months after exposure to hepatitis C virus (HCV) are regarded as acute hepatitis C.
- Two patient populations worldwide share the highest prevalence of acute HCV infection: injection drug users and HIV-positive men who have sex with men.
- Diagnosis of acute HCV is often difficult in both patient populations because the acute inflammatory phase can be asymptomatic and patients at highest risk for acquiring acute HCV (injection drug users) tend to evade regular medical care.

INTRODUCTION

The first 6 months after exposure to hepatitis C virus (HCV) are regarded as acute hepatitis C (AHC).[1,2] Two patient populations worldwide share the highest prevalence of AHC virus infection: injection drug users and HIV-positive men who have sex with men (MSM). Within the latter a substantial increase in AHC cases has been observed over the past decade. Diagnosis of AHC is often difficult in both patient populations because the acute inflammatory phase can be clinically asymptomatic and patients at highest risk for acquiring AHC (injection drug users) tend to evade regular medical care. Type and duration of treatment vary depending on the presence of an auxiliary HIV infection. This article addresses similarities and differences in the epidemiology, diagnosis, and management of AHC monoinfection and coinfection.

a Department of Internal Medicine I, Bonn University Hospital, Sigmund-Freud-Straße 25, 53105 Bonn, Germany; b Department of Gastroenterology, Hepatology and Endocrinology, Hannover Medical School, Carl-Neuberg Str. 1, 30625 Hannover, Germany
* Corresponding author.
E-mail address: juergen.rockstroh@ukb.uni-bonn.de

Infect Dis Clin N Am 26 (2012) 995–1010
http://dx.doi.org/10.1016/j.idc.2012.08.011
0891-5520/12/$ – see front matter © 2012 Elsevier Inc. All rights reserved.

id.theclinics.com

EPIDEMIOLOGY

The highest prevalence and incidence of AHC monoinfection in developed countries can be found in injection drug users.[3–12] Other risk factors include blood transfusion from unscreened donors, unsafe therapeutic injections, and other health care–related procedures (**Table 1**).[13–16] Mother-to-child transmission of HCV has also been reported but on a very infrequent basis (see **Table 1**).[14]

Sexual intercourse with HCV-positive partners or promiscuity has been reported as a likely risk factor for acquiring HCV infection in 22% of cases in the German Hep-Net Acute HCV Studies I–III including more than 250 patients.[17] However, overall sexual transmission of HCV in serodiscordant heterosexual couples has been rare, with a lifetime risk less than 1% (see **Table 1**).[18,19] Still, reported sexual transmissions of HCV have been increasing in a U.S. report on acute HCV.[15] Although a history of intravenous drug abuse was still the most frequent cause for HCV infection in 48% of cases, 42% of the participants reported more than one sex partner and 10% revealed their sexual preference as MSM. The broader availability of lifestyle drugs, such as sildenafil, and use of noninjecting drugs has influenced sexual culture and has been shown to significantly increase the risk for HIV and other sexually transmitted diseases, not only in MSM but also in other populations.[20–23]

Nevertheless, most sexually transmitted acute HCV infections worldwide have been reported among HIV-positive MSM (**Fig. 1**).[16,24–51] These cases of AHC seemed to be linked to unsafe sex and recreational drug use, particularly sexual practices with high risk for blood–blood contact, including fisting, unprotected anal sex, and nasal snorting of drugs, which were previously considered rare and inefficient transmission routes.[52] This overlapping of risk factors may also be an important aspect in transmitting AHC infection via the sexual route. Within the German behavioral study,[52] 30% of patients with sexually transmitted AHC infection reported 2 or 3 risk factors, compared with 6% of controls.

Furthermore, transmission seems to occur via social networks separate from intravenous drug use. Phylogenetic analyses identified MSM-specific clustering of HCV strains, with almost three-quarters of HCV strains found in Europe circulating in more than one country. Viral sequences from injection drug users or endemic HCV strains were not part of any of these clusters.[53,54] Additionally, phylogenetic analyses of the Australian Trial in Acute Hepatitis C (ATAHC), in which a significant proportion of MSM self-reported intravenous drug abuse was the most likely route of hepatitis C

Table 1 Average estimated risk of transmission for HIV, HCV, and HIV/HCV coinfection			
Mode of Transmission	HIV	HCV	HIV/HCV
Perinatal	10%–20%	<2%–7%	10%–20%
Sexual contact	<1%	<1%	<1%–3%[a]
Needle stick injury with cannula	0.3%	0.4%	Unknown

[a] Values are based from data from HCV serodiscordant heterosexual couples. It has to be speculated that, within the current outbreak of HCV in MSM, traumatic mucosal damage through unprotected anal sex or fisting with high risk of blood–blood contacts, the risk for acquisition of HCV is much higher.

Modified from Lacombe K, Rockstroh JK. HIV and viral hepatitis co-infections: advances and challenges. Gut 2012;61(Suppl 1):i48.

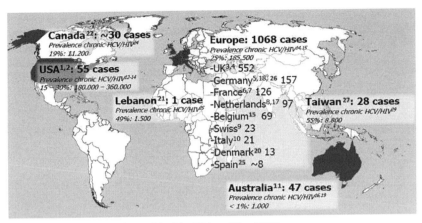

Fig. 1. Prevalence of acute hepatitis C in HIV-positive MSM.

transmission, revealed MSM-specific clustering regardless of the underlying mode of transmission.[36]

DIAGNOSIS

The AHC period is defined as the first 6 months after infection with HCV. Because the exact time point of infection is often difficult to determine, distinguishing between a true AHC and early chronic infection is frequently difficult.[1,2] Seroconversion from anti-HCV negativity to anti-HCV positivity, reflecting the development of antibodies, can be regarded as a definite diagnosis. However, because observable seroconversion is uncommon in clinical care, HCV RNA testing via polymerase chain reaction must be performed if AHC is suspected and anti-HCV antibodies are still negative. However, anti-HCV positivity does not necessarily imply a long-lasting chronic infection, but can also be observed in the acute phase. If prior serologic testing is not available (in injection drug users), viral load fluctuations and low-level viremia can be useful in distinguishing acute from chronic phase HCV infection.[55]

In addition, elevated aminotransferases can be a helpful indicator of AHC, although definitions vary from study to study. In contrast to HIV-positive patients who are seen every 3 to 6 months for routine control of HIV infection, those who are HIV-negative may consult with their general practitioner on a less frequent basis, and therefore acute liver transaminase elevations may possibly be missed in the HIV-negative population and thus only symptomatic patients are diagnosed. In addition, timely diagnosis is problematic because most individuals with acute HCV infection are asymptomatic. Only around one-third to a half of individuals with acute HCV infection show signs of an acute illness, such as lethargy and myalgia, and less frequently jaundice.[16,33] In the German Hep-Net AHC cohort, disease severity was not associated with HCV genotype, viral load, age, sex, and body mass index.[17] HIV-positive patients are less likely to experience a clinically apparent AHC infection.[16,33] In addition, anti-HCV seroconversion may be significantly delayed in HIV-positive patients, with 5% of cases still anti-HCV–negative despite ongoing viral replication for 1 year.[56] However, at least annual anti-HCV antibody and 6-monthly alanine aminotransferase (ALT) measurements followed by HCV RNA testing in cases of suspected AHC seems to be a reasonable approach for AHC screening in HIV-positive individuals.[57] This recommendation derives from findings from the British St Mary's Acute Hepatitis C Cohort (SMACC), in which 88% of patients experienced elevated ALT within 3 months of infection, with peak ALT levels greater than 5 times the upper limit of normal in 55%.[56] In the absence of consensus recommendations, screening for clinically asymptomatic AHC in other at-risk populations, such as HIV-negative MSM and injection drug users, should consist of at least annual anti-HCV antibody testing. HCV RNA testing may be performed after defined high-risk exposures or clinical suspicion, which would be similar to recommendations after occupational exposure, wherein HCV RNA should be tested after 2 to 4 weeks.[58]

Clinicians worldwide are beginning to notice a second wave of AHC in HIV-infected individuals who had been successfully treated for or had spontaneously cleared their first episode of AHC previously.[59–61] This area clearly needs further study to identify risk factors for reinfection.

Natural Course

Rates of spontaneous HCV clearance have been estimated as high as 25% of cases in AHC monoinfection.[62] In some special cohorts, such young women, even up to 50% of patients may clear the virus without any antiviral treatment.[63] In contrast, chronicity rates are high in HIV-coinfected individuals, with around 85% of patients experiencing progression to chronic hepatitis C.[35,56,64–67] Scientific interest is still high in identifying predictors of viral clearance, because this would allow clinicians to expose to antiviral therapy only those patients who would not clear HCV spontaneously. Unfortunately, most of these studies lack power because of the number of patients evaluated is too small to accurately distinguish between predictive factors. So far, factors associated with spontaneous HCV clearance include symptomatic disease, female gender, nonblack ethnicity, clearance of HCV RNA within 4 weeks after onset of clinical symptoms, presence of neutralizing antibodies, T-cell responses, natural killer (NK) cell activities and the presence of distinct NK cell receptor and HLA ligands, hepatitis B surface antigen (HBsAg) positivity, and geographic region (other European regions vs southern Europe/Argentina).[68–84] Additionally, 2 studies have described high ALT and CD4 cell count as predictors for spontaneous clearance in HIV coinfection.[66,85]

In recent years, genome-wide association studies in HCV monoinfection identified single nucleotide polymorphisms (SNP) near the IL28B gene encoding for interferon lambda that constitute a crucial part of the host's innate immune defense against HCV.[66,84–89] Individuals with the CC genotype of the SNP rs12979860 were more than 3 times as likely to clear HCV RNA as individuals with CT and TT genotypes.[64,87,88,90] The IL28B genotype seems to be less important in patients with jaundice.[91] Similar observations regarding the influence of IL28B on spontaneous clearance rates have been made in HIV/HCV coinfected individuals.[37,48] These SNPs could explain differences in spontaneous clearance rates between races, because the frequency of the protective allele varies across ethnic groups, with a lower frequency in those of African origin compared with European patients.[87] The role of different SNPs in the IL28B region is currently a matter of debate. A positive impact of 4 SNPs, rs8099917 TT, rs8105790 TT, rs12980275 AA, and rs10853728 CC, on spontaneous clearance of HCV was shown in an Asian cohort infection.[92] In this cohort no link was seen between the rs12979860 SNP and spontaneous clearance of HCV infection. Further studies are needed to clarify the value of IL28b genotyping in AHC and whether treatment decisions can be based on distinct SNPs in the Il28b gene.[93]

To date, inconclusive data exist on liver fibrosis progression after AHC in HIV coinfection. Cohort data from the United States showed moderately advanced fibrosis on liver biopsy of 82% of patients (n = 11) with higher age, longer duration of HIV infection, and longer exposure to antiretroviral therapy.[94] Additionally, recent data from the European AHC Cohort should reassure patients and clinicians about the risk of liver cirrhosis after AHC, because the investigators found no evidence of a fastened fibrosis progression rate, assessed mainly with transelastography, in 45 patients over a median follow-up of 6 months after diagnosis of AHC.[95]

To further investigate into the epidemiology, natural history, and treatment outcomes of acute HCV infection in a more meaningful setting, the European AIDS Treatment Network (NEAT) group recently opened a multicenter prospective cohort study for recruitment, in which 600 HIV-positive and HIV-negative patients with documented AHC infection will be followed prospectively over an initial period of 3 years after diagnosis of AHC infection (PROBE-C study; ClinicalTrials.gov identifier: NCT01289652).

START OF TREATMENT

Also of high clinical significance is the determination of the point in time until which spontaneous clearance can be expected and subsequent treatment can be postponed without impeding its efficacy. In AHC monoinfection, early treatment is usually advisable, but so far no consensus exists. In patients who do not seem to be spontaneous clearers 2 to 4 months after onset of AHC, antiviral treatment should be considered, because 80% to 90% of patients may respond to interferon monotherapy.[1] Researchers have also suggested following these patients with HCV RNA quantification every 4 weeks and treating only those still positive at 12 weeks after initial presentation.[93] Data from a small cohort in HIV-negative patients support the definition of 12 weeks' HCV RNA negativity as a predictor of chronicity.[96] In this study, only 2 of 24 cases with spontaneous clearance had HCV RNA detectable 12 weeks after diagnosis, and none did after 16 weeks. However, some clinicians may prefer to start treatment earlier if the HCV RNA is persistently high.[1] Recent data from the German Hep-Net Acute HCV III study, to date the largest and first randomized European trial on AHC, confirm that early immediate treatment with pegylated interferon α-2b (PEG-IFNα-2b) is highly effective in both symptomatic and asymptomatic patients, and that delayed PEG-IFNα-2b plus ribavirin treatment may result in lower overall response rates in symptomatic patients in the absence of good adherence.[97] An economic evaluation in this patient population showed that early monotherapy was more cost-effective.[98] An algorithm for the treatment of AHC monoinfection is shown in **Fig. 2**.

In HIV/AHC coinfection, several cohort data have provided useful answers to the question of whether progression to chronicity of AHC infection can be predicted by looking at the course of HCV RNA after diagnosis. In a European cohort of 92 HIV-positive patients with acute HCV who did not receive HCV-specific antiviral therapy, the sensitivity and specificity of HCV RNA determination for predicting the outcome of AHC were similarly strong 4 and 12 weeks after diagnosis.[99,100] Nine of 10 patients showing spontaneous regression of HCV RNA of at least 2 log 4 weeks after diagnosis subsequently cleared HCV, whereas 92% of patients who were HCV RNA–positive 12 weeks after diagnosis developed chronic HCV. Further support comes again from the SMACC cohort, in which a rapid decline in HCV RNA (>2 log within 100 days of infection) in 112 HIV-infected patients was also identified as a predictor for spontaneous clearance, along with high CD4 T-cell count and elevated bilirubin and ALT levels.[66]

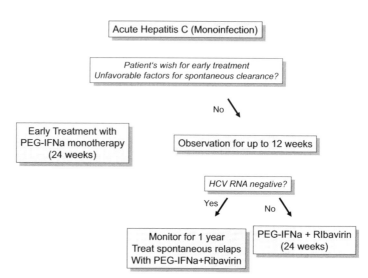

Fig. 2. Algorithm for the treatment of AHC monoinfection.

Comfortingly, a delay of 12 weeks in starting antiviral therapy has been shown to not impair the virologic outcome; the ATAHC cohort showed that treatment response rates seemed similar in AHC or early chronic HCV infection in both HIV-negative and HIV-positive patients.[101]

In the light of the given data, experts such as the European AIDS Treatment Network (NEAT) acute HCV consensus panel recommend that treatment be offered to all HIV patients who do not spontaneously show a drop in HCV RNA of more than 2 log at week 4 or who are still HCV RNA–positive at week 12 after diagnosis (**Fig. 3**).[57]

Type of Treatment

Over the years, reports of cohorts studying treatment of AHC in HIV-negative and HIV-positive individuals have accumulated.

In AHC monoinfection, high sustained virologic response (SVR; undetectable HCV RNA 24 weeks after end of treatment) rates up to 90% or even higher regardless of HCV genotype have been reported with PEG-IFNα monotherapy.[96,102–104] The study by Wiegand and colleagues[96] also highlights the importance of adherence to therapy for successful treatment responses in populations with mediocre compliance. The low overall SVR rate of 71% could be explained as reflecting a substantial proportion of nonadherent patients. Among those adherent to therapy, the SVR rate was 89%. The usual treatment of AHC should therefore be based on PEG-IFNα monotherapy (ie, either PEG-IFNα-2a, 180 μg/wk, or PEG-IFNα-2b, 1.5 μg/kg/wk).[1] Combination therapy with ribavirin does not significantly increase the SVR rate but may be considered in those patients in whom the differential diagnosis of acute versus chronic hepatitis is uncertain.[1] In the German Hep-Net Acute HCV III study, delayed PEG-IFNα-2b plus ribavirin treatment in symptomatic patients fully adherent to therapy led to response rates similar to those seen with early immediate treatment with PEG-IFNα-2b monotherapy.[97] To date, data supporting the addition of ribavirin to PEG-IFN in the treatment of early AHC monoinfection are still inconclusive.[105] In clinical practice, starting monotherapy with PEG-IFN and monitoring HCV RNA may be reasonable. If

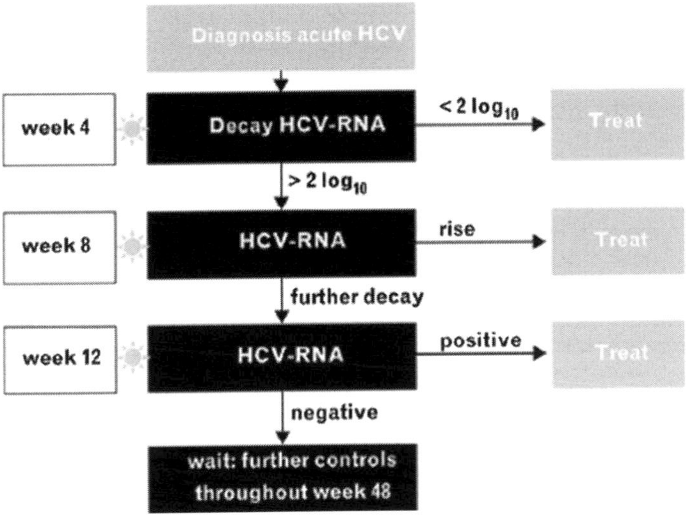

Fig. 3. Starting antiviral therapy according to the course of HCV RNA in HIV coinfection. (*Reproduced from* Deterding K, Gruner NH, Buggisch P, et al. Early versus delayed treatment of acute hepatitis C: the German HEP-NET Acute HCV-III study - a randomized controlled trial. Presented at the 47th Annual Meeting of the European Association for the Study of the Liver (EASL 2012). Barcelona, Spain, April 18–22, 2012; with permission.)

patients do not become HCV RNA–negative by week 4, the addition of ribavirin should be considered.

In AHC coinfection, SVR rates of 60% to 80% after early antiviral therapy with PEG-IFN and ribavirin have been shown within clinical studies and cohorts, regardless of HCV genotype.[24,49,50,85,106–111] These rates are clearly higher compared with those observed in the setting of chronic HCV infection, wherein rates of around 30% are reached for genotype 1 infection,[112,113] which is the predominant HCV genotype in acute HCV infection. Patients were treated with PEG-IFNs at standard doses (PEG-IFNα-2b, 1.5 µg/kg/wk, and PEG-IFNα-2a, 180 µg/wk), and ribavirin was used in 85% of patients.

The added value of ribavirin is still very much a focus of scientific interest. Ribavirin nonetheless seems to be necessary to reach high response rates in HIV-coinfected patients in light of case reports of inefficient PEG-IFN monotherapy from Germany[106] and a first pilot trial of PEG-IFN monotherapy from the Netherlands.[37] In addition, riba-virin's important contribution to improving viral kinetic response has been shown in early chronic infection in the aforementioned ATAHC study in which greater reductions in HCV RNA were seen between weeks 8 and 12 of treatment in HIV/HCV coinfected patients receiving combination therapy compared with PEG-IFN alone in monoin-fected patients.[114,115]

With regard to IL28B's influence on treatment outcome, published data from a German cohort showed that, in contrast to HIV-infected patients with chronic HCV, the IL28B genotype was not significantly associated with treatment response rates in patients with AHC,[38,116] which is in line with known data on the effect of IL28B in the treatment of AHC in HIV-negative individuals.[64,93]

To date, no data exist on the efficacy and safety of specifically targeted antiviral therapy for HCV genotype 1 with the novel HCV protease inhibitors in the setting of acute HCV monoinfection or coinfection.

Duration of Treatment

The usual duration of treatment in AHC monoinfection is 24 weeks.[1,117] A small number of studies have evaluated different short-course therapies (8, 12 weeks) but failed to show similar SVR rates, as seen after 24 weeks of treatment.[118–124] The only independent factor associated with SVR was a rapid virologic response (RVR; undetectable HCV RNA at week 4 of treatment).

Analogous to using viral kinetics in predicting spontaneous viral clearance, evidence for the use of viral kinetics in determining the chance of SVR and potentially the optimal length of therapy in AHC coinfection comes from the European multicenter cohort study.[119] In this observational cohort, patients who were able to achieve a viral load of less than 600 IU/mL at week 4 had a very high chance of reaching SVR. In contrast, therapy was likely to fail in patients who did not reach a viral load of less than 600 IU/mL at week 12. An additional subanalysis showed that German patients who were treated for at least 20 weeks or longer after a first HCV RNA level of less than 600 IU/mL had a 96% chance of cure (SVR), compared with only 20% of patients reached SVR if they were treated less than 20 weeks after a first HCV RNA level of less than 600 IU/mL.[119] Although 48 weeks of therapy for acute HCV in HIV-infected patients seemed more efficacious than 24 weeks in another single study,[120] other reports in AHC coinfection showed SVR rates of greater than 70%, with no statistically significant difference by length of therapy.[101,106,121] Most recent data from the United Kingdom support the RVR-driven treatment duration, as recommended by the NEAT consensus panel.[57,122,125]

Modern commercial assays have reached lower limits of HCV RNA detection of 10 or 15 IU/mL. Although the value of more sensitive assays for defining virologic response have not yet been explored in the setting of acute HCV infection, residual viremia less than 600 IU/mL at week 4 of treatment has been associated with decreased odds for achieving SVR in the setting of chronic HCV infection.[123]

In summary, experts recommend using PEG-IFN and weight-based ribavirin for all HIV-positive patients with AHC infection. Stopping ribavirin after week 12 in patients who have achieved a negative HCV RNA level at week 8 or 12 may be an option for those experiencing ribavirin-associated toxicity. Viral decay may be slowed in HIV-positive compared with HIV-negative patients, and groups of patients may benefit from prolonged duration of treatment. The NEAT Acute Hepatitis C Infection Consensus Panel therefore recommends considering 24 weeks of therapy sufficient if patients reach RVR; in patients who do not reach RVR, 48 weeks may be considered (**Fig. 4**).[57]

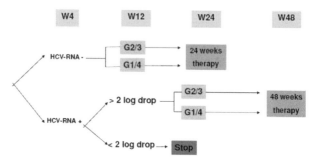

Fig. 4. Duration of antiviral therapy according to the course of HCV RNA in HIV coinfection.

SUMMARY

Transmission of HCV mainly occurs in injection drugs users and HIV-positive individuals, especially MSM, in whom AHC has been increasing over the past decade. The rates of spontaneous viral clearance are estimated at around 15% for HIV-positive and 25% for HIV-negative individuals. Early antiviral therapy is recommended in patients who do not reach a significant decay of HCV RNA 4 weeks after diagnosis or who still have detectable HCV RNA 12 weeks after diagnosis. The current standard regimen for treating acute HCV infection is PEG-IFN for 24 weeks in HIV-negative individuals regardless of HCV genotype, and PEG-IFN in combination with weight-based ribavirin in HIV-positive individuals. Duration of treatment should be adjusted based on the initial virologic response to antiviral therapy. Randomized controlled trials are urgently needed to help develop guidelines on best clinical management of AHC, including topics such as use of newly developed protease inhibitors, added value of ribavirin, and influence of HCV genotype and IL28B genotype polymorphism on treatment duration.

REFERENCES

1. European Association for the Study of the Liver. EASL Clinical Practice Guidelines: management of hepatitis C virus infection. J Hepatol 2011;55(2):245–64.
2. Ghany MG, Strader DB, Thomas DL, et al. Diagnosis, management, and treatment of hepatitis C: an update. Hepatology 2009;49(4):1335–74.
3. Robotin MC, Copland J, Tallis G, et al. Surveillance for newly acquired hepatitis C in Australia. J Gastroenterol Hepatol 2004;19:283–8.
4. Wu HX, Wu J, Wong T, et al. Enhanced surveillance of newly acquired hepatitis C virus infection in Canada, 1998 to 2004. Scand J Infect Dis 2006;38:482–9.
5. Rantala M, van de Laar MJ. Surveillance and epidemiology of hepatitis B and C in Europe—a review. Euro Surveill 2008;13:18880.
6. Armstrong GL, Wasley A, Simard EP, et al. The prevalence of hepatitis C virus infection in the United States, 1999 through 2002. Ann Intern Med 2006;144:705–14.
7. Mele A, Tosti ME, Marzolini A, et al. Prevention of hepatitis C in Italy: lessons from surveillance of type-specific acute viral hepatitis. SEIEVA collaborating Group. J Viral Hepat 2000;7:30–5.
8. Patrick DM, Tyndall MW, Cornelisse PG, et al. Incidence of hepatitis C virus infection among injection drug users during an outbreak of HIV infection. CMAJ 2001;165:889–95.
9. Maher L, et al. Incidence and risk factors for hepatitis C seroconversion in injecting drug users in Australia. Addiction 2006;101:1499–508.
10. Roy E, Alary M, Morissette C, et al. High hepatitis C virus prevalence and incidence among Canadian intravenous drug users. Int J STD AIDS 2007;18:23–7.
11. Roy E, Boudreau JF, Boivin JF. Hepatitis C virus incidence among young street-involved IDUs in relation to injection experience. Drug Alcohol Depend 2009;102:158–61.
12. Grebely J, Prins M, Hellard M, et al. Hepatitis C virus clearance, reinfection, and persistence, with insights from studies of injecting drug users: towards a vaccine. Lancet Infect Dis 2012;12(5):408–14.
13. Lacombe K, Rockstroh JK. HIV and viral hepatitis co-infections: advances and challenges. Gut 2012;61(Suppl 1):i47–58.
14. Shepard CW, Finelli L, Alter MJ. Global epidemiology of hepatitis C virus infection. Lancet Infect Dis 2005;5:558–67.
15. Daniels D, Grytdal S, Wasley A. Surveillance for acute viral hepatitis—United States, 2007. MMWR Surveill Summ 2009;58:1–27.

16. Vogel M, Deterding K, Wiegand J, et al. Initial presentation of acute hepatitis C virus (HCV) infection among HIV-negative and HIV-positive individuals: experience from 2 large German networks on the study of acute HCV infection. Clin Infect Dis 2009;49:317–9 [author reply: 9].

17. Deterding K, Wiegand J, Grüner N, et al. The German Hep-Net acute hepatitis C cohort: impact of viral and host factors on the initial presentation of acute hepatitis C virus infection. Z Gastroenterol 2009;47(6):531–40.

18. Marincovich B, Castilla J, del Romero J, et al. Absence of hepatitis C virus transmission in a prospective cohort of heterosexual serodiscordant couples. Sex Transm Infect 2003;79:160–2.

19. Vandelli C, Renzo F, Romano L, et al. Lack of evidence of sexual transmission of hepatitis C among monogamous couples: results of a 10-year prospective follow-up study. Am J Gastroenterol 2004;99:855–9.

20. van de Laar TJ, Paxton WA, Zorgdrager F, et al. Sexual transmission of hepatitis C virus in human immunodeficiency virus-negative men who have sex with men: a series of case reports. Sex Transm Dis 2011;38(2):102–4.

21. Nguyen O, Sheppeard V, Douglas MW, et al. Acute hepatitis C infection with evidence of heterosexual transmission. J Clin Virol 2010;49:65–8.

22. Carey JW, Mejia R, Bingham T, et al. Drug use, high-risk sex behaviors, and increased risk for recent HIV infection among men who have sex with men in Chicago and Los Angeles. AIDS Behav 2009;13:1084–96.

23. Thiede H, Jenkins RA, Carey JW, et al. Determinants of recent HIV infection among Seattle-area men who have sex with men. Am J Public Health 2009; 99(Suppl 1):S157–64.

24. Luetkemeyer A, Hare CB, Stansell J, et al. Clinical presentation and course of acute hepatitis C infection in HIV-infected patients. J Acquir Immune Defic Syndr 2006;41:31–6.

25. Cox AL, Page K, Bruneau J, et al. Rare birds in North America: acute hepatitis C cohorts. Gastroenterology 2009;136(1):26–31.

26. Giraudon I, Ruf M, Maguire H, et al. Increase in diagnosed newly acquired hepatitis C in HIV-positive men who have sex with men across London and Brighton, 2002–2006: is this an outbreak? Sex Transm Infect 2008;84:111–5.

27. Ruf M, Cohuet S, Maguire H, et al, SNAHC Steering Group. Setting up an enhanced surveillance of newly acquired hepatitis C infection in men who have sex with men: a pilot in London and South East region of England. Euro Surveill 2008;13(47):pii.19042.

28. Gambotti L, Batisse D, Colin-de-Verdiere N, et al. Acute hepatitis C infection in HIV positive men who have sex with men in Paris, France, 2001–2004. Euro Surveill 2005;10:115–7.

29. Morin T, Pariente A, Lahmek P, et al. Favorable outcome of acute occupational hepatitis C in healthcare workers: a multicenter French study on 23 cases. Eur J Gastroenterol Hepatol 2011;23(6):515–20.

30. Urbanus AT, van de Laar TJ, Stolte IG, et al. Hepatitis C virus infections among HIV-infected men who have sex with men: an expanding epidemic. AIDS 2009; 23:F1–7.

31. Rauch A, Rickenbach M, Weber R, et al. Unsafe sex and increased incidence of hepatitis C virus infection among HIV-infected men who have sex with men: the Swiss HIV Cohort Study. Clin Infect Dis 2005;41:395–402.

32. Gallotta G, Gali L, De Bona A, et al. Acute hepatitis C virus in HIV co-infected men who have sex with men: Milan, 1996–2007. Presented at the 4th International HIV and Hepatitis Co-infection. Madrid, June 19–21, 2008.

33. Matthews G, Hellard M, Haber P, et al. Characteristics and treatment outcomes among HIV-infected individuals in the Australian Trial in Acute Hepatitis C. Clin Infect Dis 2009;48:650–8.
34. Sherman KE, Rouster SD, Horn PS. Comparison of methodologies for quantification of hepatitis C virus (HCV) RNA in patients coinfected with HCV and human immunodeficiency virus. Clin Infect Dis 2002;35(4):482–7.
35. Soriano V, Mocroft A, Rockstroh J, et al. Spontaneous viral clearance, viral load, and genotype distribution of hepatitis C virus (HCV) in HIV-infected patients with anti-HCV antibodies in Europe. J Infect Dis 2008;198:1337–44.
36. Matthews GV, Pham ST, Hellard M, et al. Patterns and characteristics of hepatitis C transmission clusters among HIV-positive and HIV-negative individuals in the Australian Trial in Acute Hepatitis C. Clin Infect Dis 2011; 52(6):803–11.
37. Arends JE, Lambers FA, van der Meer JT, et al. Treatment of acute hepatitis C virus infection in HIV+ patients: Dutch recommendations for management. Neth J Med 2011;69(1):43–9.
38. Neukam K, Nattermann J, Rallón N, et al. Different distributions of hepatitis C virus genotypes among HIV-infected patients with acute and chronic hepatitis C according to interleukin-28B genotype. HIV Med 2011;12(8):487–93.
39. Bottieau E, Apers L, Van Esbroeck M, et al. Hepatitis C virus infection in HIV-infected men who have sex with men: sustained rising incidence in Antwerp, Belgium, 2001-2009. Euro Surveill 2010;15(39):19673.
40. Barfod TS, Omland LH, Katzenstein TL. Incidence and characteristics of sexually transmitted acute hepatitis C virus infection among HIV-positive men who have sex with men in Copenhagen, Denmark during four years (2006-2009): a retrospective cohort study. Scand J Infect Dis 2011;43(2):145–8.
41. Dionne-Odom J, Osborn MK, Radziewicz H, et al. Acute hepatitis C and HIV co-infection. Lancet Infect Dis 2009;9(12):775–83.
42. Remis RA. Study to Characterize the Epidemiology of Hepatitis C Infection in Canada. 2002. Final Report. Public Health Agency of Canada. Available at: http://www.phac-aspc.gc.ca/hepc/pubs/hepc2002/index-eng.php. Accessed May 20, 2012.
43. Lebanese Republic, Ministry of Public Health. UNGASS Country Progress Report Lebanon March 2010. Available at: http://www.unaids.org/en/dataanalysis/monitoringcountryprogress/2010progressreportssubmittedbycountries/lebanon_2010_country_progress_report_en.pdf. Accessed May 20, 2012.
44. Boesecke C, Stellbrink HJ, Mauss S, et al. Does Baseline HCV Genotype Have an Impact upon Treatment Outcome of Acute HCV Infection in HIV Co-Infected Individuals? Presented at the 18th Conference on Retroviruses and Opportunistic Infections. Boston, February 27-March 2, 2011.
45. Sun HY, Chang SY, Yang TY, et al. Recent hepatitis C virus infection in HIV-positive patients in Taiwan: incissdence and risk factors. J Clin Microbiol 2012;50(3):781–7.
46. Lee HC, Ko NY, Lee NY, et al. Seroprevalence of viral hepatitis and sexually transmitted disease among adults with recently diagnosed HIV infection in Southern Taiwan, 2000-2005: upsurge in hepatitis C virus infections among injection drug users. J Formos Med Assoc 2008;107(5):404–11.
47. Larsen C, Alric L, Auperin I, et al. Acute hepatitis C in HIV-infected men who have sex with men in France in 2006 and 2007. Presented at the 58th Annual Meeting of the American Association for the Study of the Liver. Boston, November 2–6, 2007.

48. Clausen LN, Weis N, Astvad K, et al. Interleukin-28B polymorphisms are associated with hepatitis C virus clearance and viral load in a HIV-1-infected cohort. J Viral Hepat 2011;18(4):e66–74.

49. van der Helm JJ, Prins M, Del Amo J, et al. The hepatitis C epidemic among HIV-positive MSM: incidence estimates from 1990 to 2007. AIDS 2011;25(8): 1083–91.

50. Fierer D, Fishman S, Uriel A, et al. Characterization of an outbreak of acute HCV infection in HIV-infected men in New York city. Presented at the 16th Conference on Retroviruses and Opportunistic Infections. Montreal, February 8–11, 2009.

51. Hung CC, Chen MY, Hsieh SM, et al. Impact of chronic hepatitis C infection on outcomes of patients with an advanced stage of HIV-1 infection in an area of low prevalence of co-infection. Int J STD AIDS 2005;16(1):42–8.

52. Schmidt AJ, Rockstroh JK, Vogel M, et al. Trouble with bleeding: risk factors for acute hepatitis C among HIV-positive gay men from Germany–a case-control study. PLoS One 2011;6(3):e17781.

53. van de Laar T, Pybus O, Bruisten S, et al. Evidence of a large, international network of HCV transmission in HIV-positive men who have sex with men. Gastroenterology 2009;136:1609–17.

54. Vogel M, van de Laar T, Kupfer B, et al. Phylogenetic analysis of acute hepatitis C virus genotype 4 infections among human immunodeficiency virus-positive men who have sex with men in Germany. Liver Int 2010;30(8):1169–72.

55. McGovern BH, Brich CE, Bowen MJ, et al. Improving the diagnosis of acute hepatitis C virus infection with expanded viral load criteria. Clin Infect Dis 2009;24:1051–60.

56. Thomson EC, Nastouli E, Main J, et al. Delayed anti-HCV antibody response in HIV-positive men acutely infected with HCV. AIDS 2009;23:89–93.

57. The European AIDS Treatment Network (NEAT) Acute Hepatitis C Infection Consensus Panel. Acute hepatitis C in HIV-infected individuals: recommendations from the European AIDS Treatment Network (NEAT) consensus conference. AIDS 2011;25(4):399–409.

58. Kubitschke A, Bahr MJ, Aslan N, et al. Induction of hepatitis C virus (HCV)-specific T cells by needle stick injury in the absence of HCV-viraemia. Eur J Clin Invest 2007;37(1):54–64.

59. Stellbrink HJ, Schewe CK, Vogel M, et al. Increasing numbers of acute hepatitis C infections in HIV-infected MSM and high reinfection rates following SVR. J Int AIDS Soc 2010;13(Suppl 4):P200.

60. Lambers F, Prins M, Thomas X, et al. High incidence rate of HCV reinfection after treatment of acute HCV infection in HIV-infected MSM in Amsterdam. AIDS 2011;25(17):F21–7.

61. Ingiliz P, Krznaric I, Hoffmann C, et al. Prior HCV Infection Does Not Protect from Sexually Transmitted HCV Reinfection in HIV+ MSM. Presented at the 19th Conference on Retroviruses and Opportunistic Infections. Seattle, March 5–8, 2012.

62. Micallef JM, Kaldor JM, Dore GJ. Spontaneous viral clearance following acute hepatitis C infection: a systematic review of longitudinal studies. J Viral Hepat 2006;13:34–41.

63. Wiese M, Berr F, Lafrenz M, et al. Low frequency of cirrhosis in a hepatitis C (genotype 1b) single-source outbreak in germany: a 20-year multicenter study. Hepatology 2000;32(1):91–6.

64. Grebely J, Petoumenos K, Hellard M, et al, ATAHC Study Group. Potential role for interleukin-28B genotype in treatment decision-making in recent hepatitis C virus infection. Hepatology 2010;52(4):1216–24.

65. Jones L, Uriel A, Kaplan D, et al. Natural history and treatment outcome of acute hepatitis C with and without HIV co-infection in a North American cohort. Peesented at the AASLD 2008 Meeting. San Francisco, California. October 31-November 1, 2008.
66. Thomson E, Fleming VM, Main J, et al. Predicting spontaneous clearance of acute hepatitis C virus in a large cohort of HIV-1-infected men. Gut 2011;60(6):837–45.
67. Thomas DL, Astemborski J, Rai RM, et al. The natural history of hepatitis C virus infection: host, viral, and environmental factors. JAMA 2000;284:450–6.
68. Grebely J, Matthews GV, Petoumenos K, et al. Spontaneous clearance and the beneficial impact of treatment on clearance during recent hepatitis C virus infection. J Viral Hepat 2009;17:896.
69. Page K, Hahn JA, Evans J, et al. Acute hepatitis C virus infection in young adult injection drug users: a prospective study of incident infection, resolution, and reinfection. J Infect Dis 2009;200:1216–26.
70. McGovern BH, Wurcel A, Kim AY, et al. Acute hepatitis C virus infection in incarcerated injection drug users. Clin Infect Dis 2006;42:1663–70.
71. Wang CC, Krantz E, Klarquist J, et al. Acute hepatitis C in a contemporary US cohort: modes of acquisition and factors influencing viral clearance. J Infect Dis 2007;196:1474–82.
72. Diepolder HM. New insights into the immunopathogenesis of chronic hepatitis C. Antiviral Res 2009;82:103–9.
73. Post J, Ratnarajah S, Lloyd AR. Immunological determinants of the outcomes from primary hepatitis C infection. Cell Mol Life Sci 2009;66:733–56.
74. Rehermann B. Hepatitis C virus versus innate and adaptive immune responses: a tale of coevolution and coexistence. J Clin Invest 2009;119:1745–54.
75. Bowen DG, Walker CM. Adaptive immune responses in acute and chronic hepatitis C virus infection. Nature 2005;436:946–52.
76. Takaki A, Wiese M, Maertens G, et al. Cellular immune responses persist and humoral responses decrease two decades after recovery from a single-source outbreak of hepatitis C. Nat Med 2000;6:578–82.
77. Ray SC, Wang YM, Laeyendecker O, et al. Acute hepatitis C virus structural gene sequences as predictors of persistent viremia: hypervariable region 1 as a decoy. J Virol 1999;73:2938–46.
78. Farci P, Shimoda A, Coiana A, et al. The outcome of acute hepatitis C predicted by the evolution of the viral quasispecies. Science 2000;288:339–44.
79. Harfouch S, Guiguet M, Valantin MA, et al. Lack of TGF-β production by hepatitis C virus-specific T cells during HCV acute phase is associated with HCV clearance in HIV coinfection. J Hepatol 2012;56(6):1259–68.
80. Schlaphoff V, Lunemann S, Suneetha PV, et al. Dual function of the NK cell receptor 2B4 (CD244) in the regulation of HCV-specific CD8+ T cells. PLoS Pathog 2011;7(5):e1002045.
81. Schulze Zur Wiesch J, Ciuffreda D, Lewis-Ximenez L, et al. Broadly directed virus-specific CD4+ T cell responses are primed during acute hepatitis C infection, but rapidly disappear from human blood with viral persistence. J Exp Med 2012;209(1):61–75.
82. Khakoo SI, Thio CL, Martin MP, et al. HLA and NK cell inhibitory receptor genes in resolving hepatitis C virus infection. Science 2004;305(5685):872–4.
83. Stegmann KA, Björkström NK, Ciesek S, et al. Interferon α-stimulated natural killer cells from patients with acute hepatitis C virus (HCV) infection recognize HCV-infected and uninfected hepatoma cells via DNAX accessory molecule-1. J Infect Dis 2012;205(9):1351–62.

84. Santantonio T, Wiegand J, Gerlach JT. Acute hepatitis C: current status and remaining challenges. J Hepatol 2008;49(4):625–33.

85. Gilleece YC, Browne RE, Asboe D, et al. Transmission of hepatitis C virus among HIV-positive homosexual men and response to a 24-week course of pegylated interferon and ribavirin. J Acquir Immune Defic Syndr 2005;40:41–6.

86. Harris HE, Eldridge KP, Harbour S, et al. Does the clinical outcome of hepatitis C infection vary with the infecting hepatitis C virus type? J Viral Hepat 2007;14: 213–20.

87. Thomas DL, Thio CL, Martin MP, et al. Genetic variation in IL28B and spontaneous clearance of hepatitis C virus. Nature 2009;461:798–801.

88. Rauch A, Kutalik Z, Descombes P, et al. Genetic variation in IL28B is associated with chronic hepatitis C and treatment failure: a genome-wide association study. Gastroenterology 2010;138:1338–45. e1331–7.

89. Ge D, Fellay J, Thompson AJ, et al. Genetic variation in IL28B predicts hepatitis C treatment-induced viral clearance. Nature 2009;461:399–401.

90. Beinhardt S, Aberle JH, Strasser M, et al. Serum level of IP-10 increases predictive value of IL28B polymorphisms for spontaneous clearance of acute HCV infection. Gastroenterology 2012;142(1):78–85.e2.

91. Tillmann HL, Thompson AJ, Patel K, et al. A polymorphism near IL28B is associated with spontaneous clearance of acute hepatitis C virus and jaundice. Gastroenterology 2010;139:1586–92.

92. Rao HY, Sun DG, Jiang D, et al. IL28B genetic variants and gender are associated with spontaneous clearance of hepatitis C virus infection. J Viral Hepat 2012;19(3):173–81.

93. Deuffic-Burban S, Castel H, Wiegand J, et al. Immediate versus delayed treatment in patients with acute hepatitis C based on IL28B polymorphism: a model-based analysis. J Hepatol 2012;57(2):260–6.

94. Fierer DS, Uriel AJ, Carriero DC, et al. Liver fibrosis during an outbreak of acute hepatitis C virus infection in HIV-infected men: a prospective cohort study. J Infect Dis 2008;198(5):683–6.

95. Vogel M, Page E, Boesecke C, et al. Liver fibrosis progression after acute HCV infection (AHC) in HIV-positive individuals. Clin Infect Dis 2012;54(4):556–9.

96. Wiegand J, Buggisch P, Boecher W, et al. Early monotherapy with pegylated interferon alpha-2b for acute hepatitis C infection: the HEP-NET acute-HCV-II study. Hepatology 2006;43:250–6.

97. Deterding K, Gruner NH, Buggisch P, et al. Early versus delayed treatment of acute hepatitis C: the German HEP-NET Acute HCV-III study - a randomized controlled trial. Presented at the 47th Annual Meeting of the European Association for the Study of the Liver (EASL 2012). Barcelona, Spain, April 18–22, 2012.

98. Dintsios CM, Haverkamp A, Wiegand J, et al. Economic evaluation of early monotherapy versus delayed monotherapy or combination therapy in patients with acute hepatitis C in Germany. Eur J Gastroenterol Hepatol 2010;22(3):278–88.

99. Vogel M, Boesecke C, Rockstroh JK. Acute hepatitis C infection in HIV-positive patients. Curr Opin Infect Dis 2011;24(1):1–6.

100. Vogel M, Page E, Matthews G, et al. Use of week 4 HCV RNA after acute HCV infection to predict chronic HCV infection. Presented at the 17th Conference on Retroviruses and Opportunistic Infections. San Francisco, California, February 16–19, 2010.

101. Dore GJ, Hellard M, Matthews GV, et al. Effective treatment of injecting drug users with recently acquired hepatitis C virus infection. Gastroenterology 2010;138(1):123–135.e1–2.

102. Jaeckel E, Cornberg M, Wedemeyer H, et al. Treatment of acute hepatitis C with interferon alfa-2b. N Engl J Med 2001;345:1452–7.
103. Nomura H, Sou S, Tanimoto H, et al. Short-term interferon-alfa therapy for acute hepatitis C: a randomized controlled trial. Hepatology 2004;39:1213–9.
104. Santantonio T, Fasano M, Sinisi E, et al. Efficacy of a 24-week course of PEG-interferon alpha-2b monotherapy in patients with acute hepatitis C after failure of spontaneous clearance. J Hepatol 2005;42:329–33.
105. Gerlach JT, Diepolder HM, Zachoval R, et al. Acute hepatitis C: high rate of both spontaneous and treatment-induced viral clearance. Gastroenterology 2003; 125:80–8.
106. Vogel M, Nattermann J, Baumgarten A, et al. Pegylated interferon-alpha for the treatment of sexually transmitted acute hepatitis C in HIV-infected individuals. Antivir Ther 2006;11:1097–101.
107. Schnuriger A, Dominguez S, Guiguet M, et al, ANRS HC EP21 study group. Acute hepatitis C in HIV-infected patients: rare spontaneous clearance correlates with weak memory CD4 T-cell responses to hepatitis C virus. AIDS 2009; 23:2079–89.
108. Dominguez S, Ghosn J, Valantin MA, et al. Efficacy of early treatment of acute hepatitis C infection with pegylated interferon and ribavirin in HIV-infected patients. AIDS 2006;20:1157–61.
109. Kruk A. Efficacy of acute HCV treatment with peg-interferon alfa-2b and ribavirin in HIV-infected patients. Presented at the 3rd International AIDS Society Conference on HIV Pathogenesis and Treatment. Rio de Janeiro, July 24–27, 2005.
110. Serpaggi J, Chaix ML, Batisse D, et al. Sexually transmitted acute infection with a clustered genotype 4 hepatitis C virus in HIV-1-infected men and inefficacy of early antiviral therapy. AIDS 2006;20:233–40.
111. Piroth L, Larsen C, Binquet C, et al, Steering Committee of the HEPAIG Study. Treatment of acute hepatitis C in human immunodeficiency virus-infected patients: the HEPAIG study. Hepatology 2010;52(6):1915–21.
112. Nunez M, Miralles C, Berdun MA, et al. Role of weight-based ribavirin dosing and extended duration of therapy in chronic hepatitis C in HIV-infected patients: the PRESCO trial. AIDS Res Hum Retroviruses 2007;23:972–82.
113. Vogel M, Ahlenstiel G, Hintsche B, et al. The influence of HAART on the efficacy and safety of pegylated interferon and ribavirin therapy for the treatment of chronic HCV infection in HIV-positive individuals. Eur J Med Res 2010;15: 102–11.
114. Matthews G, Grebely J, Hellard M, et al. Differences in early virological decline in individuals treated within the Australian Trial in Acute HCV suggest a potential benefit for the use of ribavirin. Presented at the 45th Annual Meeting of the European Association for the Study of the Liver (EASL). Vienna, Austria, April 14–18, 2010.
115. Grebely J, Hellard M, Applegate T, et al. Virological responses during treatment for recent hepatitis C virus: potential benefit for ribavirin use in HCV/HIV co-infection. AIDS 2012;26(13):1653–61.
116. Nattermann J, Vogel M, Nischalke HD, et al. Genetic variation in IL28B and treatment-induced clearance of hepatitis C virus in HIV-positive patients with acute and chronic hepatitis C. J Infect Dis 2011;203(5):595–601.
117. Grebely J, Matthews GV, Dore GJ. Treatment of acute HCV infection. Nat Rev Gastroenterol Hepatol 2011;8(5):265–74.
118. Calleri G, Cariti G, Gaiottino F, et al. A short course of pegylated interferon-alpha in acute HCV hepatitis. J Viral Hepat 2007;14:116–21.

119. Vogel M, Dominguez S, Bhagani S, et al. Treatment of acute HCV infection in HIV-positive patients: experience from a multicentre European cohort. Antivir Ther 2010;15:267–79.

120. Lambers F, Brinkman K, Schinkel J, et al. Treatment of acute hepatitis C virus infection in HIV-infected MSM: the effect of treatment duration. AIDS 2011; 25(10):1333–6.

121. Matthews GV, Dore GJ. Optimal duration of treatment for acute hepatitis C in human immunodeficiency virus-positive individuals? Hepatology 2011;53(3): 1055–6 [author reply: 1056–7].

122. Dorward J, Garrett N, Scott D, et al. Successful treatment of acute hepatitis C virus in HIV positive patients using the European AIDS Treatment Network guidelines for treatment duration. J Clin Virol 2011;52(4):367–9.

123. Carlsson T, Quist A, Weiland O, et al. Rapid viral response and treatment outcome in genotype 2 and 3 chronic hepatitis C: comparison between two HCV RNA quantitation methods. J Med Virol 2008;80(5):803–7.

124. Wedemeyer H, Cornberg M, Wiegand J, et al. Treatment duration in acute hepatitis C: the issue is not solved yet. Hepatology 2006;44:1051–2.

125. Boesecke C, Rockstroh JK. Treatment of acute hepatitis C infection in HIV-infected patients. Curr Opin HIV AIDS 2011;6(4):278–84.

Index

Note: Page numbers of article titles are in **boldface** type

Infect Dis Clin N Am 26 (2012) 1011–1021
http://dx.doi.org/10.1016/S0891-5520(12)00111-0
0891-5520/12/$ – see front matter © 2012 Elsevier Inc. All rights reserved.

id.theclinics.com

United States Postal Service

Statement of Ownership, Management, and Circulation
(All Periodicals Publications Except Requestor Publications)

1. Publication Title
Infectious Disease Clinics of North America

2. Publication Number
0 0 1 - 5 5 5 6

3. Filing Date
9/14/12

4. Issue Frequency
Mar, Jun, Sep, Dec

5. Number of Issues Published Annually
4

6. Annual Subscription Price
$271.00

7. Complete Mailing Address of Known Office of Publication (Not printer) (Street, city, county, state, and ZIP+4®)

Elsevier Inc.
360 Park Avenue South
New York, NY 10010-1710

Contact Person
Stephen R. Bushing

Telephone (Include area code)
215-239-3688

8. Complete Mailing Address of Headquarters or General Business Office of Publisher (Not printer)

Elsevier Inc., 360 Park Avenue South, New York, NY 10010-1710

9. Full Names and Complete Mailing Addresses of Publisher, Editor, and Managing Editor (Do not leave blank)

Publisher (Name and complete mailing address)

Kim Murphy, Elsevier, Inc., 1600 John F. Kennedy Blvd. Suite 1800, Philadelphia, PA 19103-2899

Editor (Name and complete mailing address)

Stephanie Donley, Elsevier, Inc., 1600 John F. Kennedy Blvd. Suite 1800, Philadelphia, PA 19103-2899

Managing Editor (Name and complete mailing address)

Sarah Barth, Elsevier, Inc., 1600 John F. Kennedy Blvd. Suite 1800, Philadelphia, PA 19103-2899

10. Owner (Do not leave blank. If the publication is owned by a corporation, give the name and address of the corporation immediately followed by the names and addresses of all stockholders owning or holding 1 percent or more of the total amount of stock. If not owned by a corporation, give the names and addresses of the individual owners. If owned by a partnership or other unincorporated firm, give its name and address as well as those of each individual owner. If the publication is published by a nonprofit organization, give its name and address.)

Full Name	Complete Mailing Address
Wholly owned subsidiary of	1600 John F. Kennedy Blvd., Ste. 1800
Reed/Elsevier, US holdings	Philadelphia, PA 19103-2899

11. Known Bondholders, Mortgagees, and Other Security Holders Owning or Holding 1 Percent or More of Total Amount of Bonds, Mortgages, or Other Securities. If none, check box ☐ None

Full Name	Complete Mailing Address
N/A	

12. Tax Status (For completion by nonprofit organizations authorized to mail at nonprofit rates) (Check one)
The purpose, function, and nonprofit status of this organization and the exempt status for federal income tax purposes:
☐ Has Not Changed During Preceding 12 Months
☐ Has Changed During Preceding 12 Months (Publisher must submit explanation of change with this statement)

PS Form 3526, September 2007 (Page 1 of 3) (Instructions Page 3)) PSN 7530-01-000-9931 **PRIVACY NOTICE:** See our Privacy policy in www.usps.com

---

13. Publication Title
Infectious Disease Clinics of North America

14. Issue Date for Circulation Data Below
September 2012

15. Extent and Nature of Circulation

			Average No. Copies Each Issue During Preceding 12 Months	No. Copies of Single Issue Published Nearest to Filing Date
a.	Total Number of Copies (Net press run)		1040	1002
b. Paid Circulation (By Mail and Outside the Mail)	(1)	Mailed Outside-County Paid Subscriptions Stated on PS Form 3541. (Include paid distribution above nominal rate, advertiser's proof copies, and exchange copies)	581	523
	(2)	Mailed In-County Paid Subscriptions Stated on PS Form 3541 (Include paid distribution above nominal rate, advertiser's proof copies, and exchange copies)		
	(3)	Paid Distribution Outside the Mails Including Sales Through Dealers and Carriers, Street Vendors, Counter Sales, and Other Paid Distribution Outside USPS®	166	179
	(4)	Paid Distribution by Other Classes Mailed Through the USPS (e.g. First-Class Mail®)		
c.	Total Paid Distribution (Sum of 15b (1), (2), (3), and (4))	▶	747	702
d. Free or Nominal Rate Distribution (By Mail and Outside the Mail)	(1)	Free or Nominal Rate Outside-County Copies Included on PS Form 3541	69	70
	(2)	Free or Nominal Rate In-County Copies Included on PS Form 3541		
	(3)	Free or Nominal Rate Copies Mailed at Other Classes Through the USPS (e.g. First-Class Mail)		
	(4)	Free or Nominal Rate Distribution Outside the Mail (Carriers or other means)		
e.	Total Free or Nominal Rate Distribution (Sum of 15d (1), (2), (3) and (4))	▶	69	70
f.	Total Distribution (Sum of 15c and 15e)	▶	816	772
g.	Copies not Distributed (See instructions to publishers #4 (page 4/5))	▶	224	230
h.	Total (Sum of 15f and g)	▶	1040	1002
i.	Percent Paid (15c divided by 15f times 100)		91.54%	90.93%

16. Publication of Statement of Ownership
☐ If the publication is a general publication, publication of this statement is required. Will be printed
in the **December 2011** issue of this publication. ☐ Publication not required.

17. Signature and Title of Editor, Publisher, Business Manager, or Owner

Stephen R. Bushing — Inventory Distribution Coordinator

Date September 14, 2012

I certify that all information furnished on this form is true and complete. I understand that anyone who furnishes false or misleading information on this form or who omits material or information requested on the form may be subject to criminal sanctions (including fines and imprisonment) and/or civil sanctions (including civil penalties).

PS Form 3526, September 2007 (Page 2 of 3)

Moving?

Make sure your subscription moves with you!

To notify us of your new address, find your **Clinics Account Number** (located on your mailing label above your name), and contact customer service at:

Email: journalscustomerservice-usa@elsevier.com

800-654-2452 (subscribers in the U.S. & Canada)
314-447-8871 (subscribers outside of the U.S. & Canada)

Fax number: 314-447-8029

Elsevier Health Sciences Division
Subscription Customer Service
3251 Riverport Lane
Maryland Heights, MO 63043

Printed and bound by CPI Group (UK) Ltd, Croydon, CR0 4YY

13/10/2024

01773590-0001